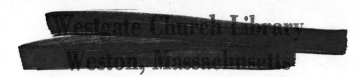
Greater Health—God's Way

SEVEN STEPS TO HEALTH, YOUTHFULNESS AND VITALITY

by

Stormie Omartian

SPARROW PRESS

1984

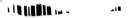

Published March 1984 by **SPARROW PRESS** of California
Canoga Park, California

Printed in the United States

ISBN: 0-917143-00-0

This book is dedicated to Diane Kendrick, my wonderful friend and secretary, for whose loving and unwavering support and assistance I am eternally grateful. I also offer special thanks to my husband, Michael, for his encouragement and willingness to give so much of himself to me and our children in order that this book could be completed.

After the book was out of my hands, Ruth Edone, my wonderful editor, brought grammatical perfection to the work. Words I had misspelled all my life were corrected and commas I had never even dreamed of were put in their proper place. Billy Ray Hearn, B. Charlyne Hinesley and Bob Angelotti did all the hard work required to put together a quality package and place it in the hands of the readers. I am deeply thankful to them for all that they have done.

CONTENTS

FOREWORD

How do you write a book about health so that it doesn't overemphasize the physical side of things and neglect the spiritual? How do you keep it from encouraging people to take themselves too seriously? How do you keep it from becoming just another collection of personal opinions?

The answer is that you begin by seeking the Lord with all your heart, and you pray continuously for guidance and wisdom and revelation. You pray for all the doors to shut on your ideas if they are not what the Lord intends. You pray for every person who hears or reads your words to be opened to what they need to know. You pray to bring life where there might be death.

My most important goal in writing this book is to convince you that God's ways are good. In fact, they are more than good. They are perfect. We experience needless pain and misery only because we do not follow His ways.

I sincerely hope that this book will whet your appetite for more knowledge and that you will want to study further on your own. At the end of this book you will find a list of books that I recommend for further reading. I have read hundreds of books on the subject of health over the last fifteen years. Many were good in some areas but poor in others, or their spiritual leanings were such that I could never recommend them. However, *all* the books I have recommended here are excellent and I encourage you to read as many of them as you can. They are consistent and solid in their overall perspective, but they do not always agree with each other on minor points. You may find that you don't agree with them on every point. That's fine—all of us may have our own opinions, each for very good reasons. Some things we can know for certain, but other things must be left to individual preference. You will need to judge each book for yourself.

Remember that this book is not a compendium of medical advice, but rather an aid to help you achieve and maintain good health. If you are sick, allow God and a doctor to help you get well. You can read this book while you are recovering and decide how you are going to change your ways.

INTRODUCTION TO THE SEVEN STEPS

Content at Any Age

When we say that everyone wants to be youthful we don't mean that if you are forty you want to look twenty, or if you are twenty you want to look ten. But if you are forty you don't want to look fifty. There is nothing wrong with being fifty and looking fifty when you *are* fifty. What *is* wrong, is being fifty and looking and feeling sixty-five. In other words, we don't want to be *prematurely* old. "Looking old" means looking older than you really are.

Every age is good. Every age has something wonderful and special about it that no other age has. Don't ever dread getting older. At any birthday you can be healthy, youthful, attractive, and alive. It's premature aging that should be unacceptable to you because premature aging is a sign that something is out of balance in your life. You may suffer under too much stress; too little exercise; a poor diet; sleepless nights; insufficient water, fresh air, sunshine, or fasting. The result will be a buildup of toxic wastes in your body that accelerates the aging process.

Because every age has its advantages, we don't want to go into our later years too decayed, decrepit, and diseased to enjoy them. To have a long and fulfilling life requires good health and an abundance of love, peace, and joy. We want to finish our lives as strong, vital, ministering people who bring good news and blessings to others. We want to be constructive, productive, contributing people. We want to be healthy, youthful, attractive, and alive, not sickly, old, repulsive, and half-dead.

Ask anyone who is sick and dying a miserable slow death how they would rather have spent their final years. They will say, "I wish I had known years ago the right way to live." Or if they have heard of the right way to live, they will say, "I wish I had listened."

Sophia, the week before she died of the cancer that had ravaged her entire body, told me, "I regret that I did not learn to forgive and release all things to God." Years of unforgiveness took its toll on Sophia and she was dead at age fifty.

Mary, after being healed of cancer of the lungs, throat, and mouth, continued against her doctor's orders to smoke, drink, and eat the way she always had. She died a very painful and sad death. She refused to follow what she knew to be the right way to live.

Max, after years of living his own way—eating junk food and being overweight, undernourished, overworked, and underexercised—decided one day that the following week he would begin a healthful diet-and-exercise program. Unfortunately, the decision came too late. The next morning he was dead of a heart attack at age forty. He had waited too long.

Ricky, a young man who practically lived on candy bars, cakes, cookies, and sodas as a regular diet, contracted leukemia. Because of the way he had fed his body, he had no resistance to help the doctors in the fight to save his life. He was dead at age twenty-five.

These are all extreme examples that began simply as premature aging. I knew all of these people personally and I watched them die needless premature deaths because either they weren't sufficiently acquainted with God's ways or they were aware of His ways and refused to follow them.

People who live in tune with God's ways and see them as good become healthy, youthful, attractive, and alive. Those who view their body as a dwelling place for the Holy Spirit of God, and, accordingly, treat it with respect and care, are best able to adapt to God's ways.

Don't be fooled by those people who always seem to do as they please with regard to their health, the ones who consume all the fast foods, junk foods, dead foods, coffee, alcohol, and cigarettes they want. They overwork and never get any exercise, fresh air, or sunshine, and they have never given a thought to fasting. Their healthy days are numbered. For people like that, retribution comes suddenly and sometimes severely. We can't disobey God's natural laws forever and get away with it. No one can. God is no respecter of persons. It doesn't matter if you have the number-one album on the Gospel record charts or have led the entire state of Maine to the Lord, if you disobey God's laws for your life and health you will have to pay the consequences.

If you have been born with a healthy, strong body, rejoice, thank God, and keep reading to find out how to keep it that way. Don't wait until something bad happens to start a diet-and-exercise program. Even if you feel good now, neglect of your health will catch up with you. Don't wait until then to find out what to do—follow the Seven Steps to Greater Health now and reap the wonderful benefits of being healthy, youthful, attractive, and alive.

An Honest Look at Yourself

Are you happy with what you see when you look in the mirror? How do your eyes look? Are they bloodshot? Dull? Tired? Swollen? Sad? Small? Tense? Lifeless? Do they burn or itch? Is your vision blurred?

What about your skin? Is it dry? Oily? Blemished? Colorless? Puffy? Grayish? Sagging? Drawn?

What about your body? Is it weak? Tired? Flabby? Overweight? Underweight? Sick? Stiff? Full of aches and pains? Do you sleep well? Do you have problems with digestion? Constipation? Frequent colds? Numerous and nameless allergies? Do you feel you're aging rapidly?

Consider your attitude. Are you depressed much of the time? Do you regret the past, curse the present, and dread the future? Do you live with feelings of bitterness, resentment, envy, rage, hopelessness, fear, or futility? Does your life seem dull? Are you lethargic or lazy? Do you have no energy?

If any of this describes you, you need to be aware that this is not the way God intended you to live and that He has provided a way out.

You see, I once suffered from almost all the maladies listed here. But I don't live with any of those problems now. I've found a way that works. It's God's way. The Seven Steps to Greater Health in this book are the steps God taught me, and I'd like to share them with you. They've worked consistently in my life for years and I've seen them work in countless other lives.

Over the Hill and Back Again

I am now forty years old, but forty is not the oldest I have ever been. The oldest I have ever been in my life was twenty-eight. I'm going to tell you what the Lord taught me that caused me to go from an old, old twenty-eight to a younger-than-ever forty.

I've got more energy and stamina than I've ever had in my life. I have overcome bad skin, bleeding gums, poor eyesight, nervous exhaustion, overweight, underweight, falling hair, lack of strength, chronic fatigue, susceptibility to constant colds and infections, menstrual problems, migraine headaches, and severely debilitating depressions. If I can overcome this poor quality of life, so can you.

I was sickly from the time I was a baby and I lived under great stress for the first twenty-eight years of my life. I know what it is like never to feel good, to be in pain, to live on tranquilizers, to face each day with feelings of futility and hopelessness, to feel that death would be better than life, to have serious diseases and then be allergic to the medicines usually used to treat them, to be sick for every important occasion that occurred in my life, to live in confusion about what was good for me and what wasn't, and to be totally ignorant of God's wonderful ways.

Now, at forty, I know what it's like to feel great, to have energy and enthusiasm, to look forward to each day, not to be sick, to have thick hair, unblemished skin, clear eyes, and to maintain a good weight. I used to be too weak to exercise; now I teach exercise classes.

When I was in my early twenties I moved to Hollywood to begin my television career as a singer, and I started taking dance lessons three times a week. I soon found I was working constantly; it was a struggle because I was often sick and always tired. The exercise I was getting in the dance classes was doing great things for my appearance, but I still suffered from physical ailments. I ate poorly, and my sleeping patterns were a joke. I would stay up all night partying, drinking, and smoking, and during the day I either slept or worked in the television studios from dawn until late at night. I never saw the sun, and I never gave a thought to fresh air or nutrition. I had a self-destructive craving for chocolate and I made sure my habit was well-fed. It's amazing how we can live so far away from God and His ways and not even see for a moment how we are destroying ourselves — we go our own way and then curse God because we feel terrible all the time. What ignorance we live in!

Finally I hit one of my all-time physical lows. I was working on the "Glen Campbell Show" from Monday through Thursday, and on a local television show from Friday through Sunday. That meant a seven-day work week. I was too insecure to turn down work, so I accepted every job I could possibly fit into my schedule. I was not obeying any of the Seven Steps to Greater Health — not one! I was headed for a collapse.

One of the other singers on the "Glen Campbell Show" was a handsome young man with clear skin, bright eyes, shiny hair, and a smiling, optimistic face who had a body that was strong, energetic, and never sick. He noticed my condition and began talking to me about such things as acidophilus, wheat germ, lecithin, apple-cider vinegar, desiccated liver, and brewer's yeast. I looked at him incredulously. He might as well have been talking Chinese, it all sounded so foreign. Remember, that was fifteen years ago and few people had heard about such foods at that time. Yet as I listened to this young man with the clear skin and healthy hair, two facts were obvious: he was healthy; I was sick. He obviously had something I needed.

He laid a plan out before me and asked, "What have you got to lose?" I thought it over for a few seconds while glancing in the mirror at my thinning hair, blemishes, darkly circled eyes, and colorless skin and said "How do I begin?"

He proceeded to acquaint me one step at a time with all of those wonder foods. The first item he prescribed was something I was able to pick up at a nearby health-food store. I had been suffering from a sore throat for weeks. That night I did what he told me to, and by the next morning my sore throat was gone. In twenty-four hours I had become a believer. From then on I read every book available on health foods. I bought every gadget, from a slant board to a juicer to a sprouter to a yogurt maker. I was into it, I was sold, I was devoted, I was fanatical! To my way of thinking, if a little was good, more would be better, and too much would be perfect. I knew no balance.

My hair started to grow back, I began to feel better, I was sick less often, and I saw my strength increase day by day. However, all that regular exercise and my extremely healthful way of eating (with emphasis on *extreme*) could not support me against the stress that flooded every area of my being. And my trust in occult practices such as numerology, astrology, hypnosis, and "positive thinking" were likewise crumbled under this stress.

Some time later, at twenty-eight, I hit another all-time low and became the oldest I have ever been in my life. There were very few parts of my body that were not affected. Physically, mentally, and emotionally I fell apart. Everything was gray—my skin, my eyes, my hair, my body, my mind, and my life. The only thing that didn't look gray to me was my future—it looked black.

Fortunately there was another singer with whom I had worked from time to time. She, like the young man on the "Glen Campbell Show," had a bright, clear, energetic, healthy attractiveness. But more than that she had an indefinable quality about her that was very appealing. She said, "I can see that you are not happy, so why don't you come with me and talk to my pastor? What have you got to lose?"

Where had I heard that before? Here I was again, so far down that I really didn't have anything to lose. So I did go with her to talk with the pastor. He sent me home with three books and said, "Read these books and come back in a week and tell me what you think of them." I devoured the books, one of which was the Gospel of John, from the Bible. I had never read anything like these books, and somehow I knew that what I was reading was the truth.

The following week, my friend and I went back to the pastor's office and there I received Jesus Christ as my personal Savior. I was, in every sense, "born again." The Holy Spirit of God came into my heart because I invited Him there, and he began to work life in me from the inside out. The tremendous, powerful, ever-reaching light of God began to flood into all my black and gray places, and I stepped out of the darkness in which I had dwelled my entire life. I asked God for His cleansing power to work in me, and clean He did. He shook my life in such a way that all the bad things fell out and all the good things remained. I began to learn of God's ways and to see that His ways are good. They were not only good, they were so far above man's ways they were not even to be compared. God's ways were perfect!

And so, in every area of my life, He began to show me what was right and what was wrong, what would bring good and what would bring bad, what would bring sickness and disease and what would bring health. He showed me, among all the many things I had learned about health, which things were really part of His intended ways for us and which were not. I began to learn balance.

I had known for years that physical exercise on a regular basis was a must for total health. I replaced the dance classes with exercise classes at a local gym with a good instructor. Soon I began teaching classes myself. However, I was well-aware that exercise alone could never be the total answer to health problems. I had also learned what wonderful things could happen just by putting high-quality foods into your body. But here, too, I learned that diet wasn't the only key to good health.

I began to see there were *many* different things that must be put together in proper balance to achieve consistently good health. All of these added up to seven steps — seven different elements that work together to bring about and preserve health and well-being.

God's Ways Are Good

The Bible says, "My people are destroyed for lack of knowledge." [1] How true! Sickness and premature death are commonplace, all because we have no knowledge of the Lord's ways. We live so very far from the way God intended us to live. That's why there is so much pain and sickness, so many headaches, heart attacks, bad tempers, mental illness, and just plain lack of joy. We suffer a great deal just because of our own ignorance about God's ways.

In his book *Back to Eden* Jethro Kloss says, "Man does not go astray from nature because he lacks intelligence or instinct, but because he wishes to gratify his own desires." I have no doubt that this is the reason man got away from God's ways in the first place—he wanted to gratify his own desires. That is why you or I get into health trouble today. We want to gratify our flesh more than we want to serve our God. Kloss goes on to say, "God has provided a remedy for every disease that might afflict us." It's possible that almost every disease is caused by some kind of violation of the natural laws of God. We don't obey them because we don't understand them.

There are people who do live God's way—in simple lifestyles, close to nature, loving the fresh, clean beauty of the outdoors. If you live on a farm and enjoy vegetables and fruits from the garden, water from your uncontaminated well, poultry and beef from the animals you raise, fish from your unpolluted lake, work from dawn to dusk in good physical labor, rest well at night, love the Lord, and fast and pray regularly to His glory—then you don't need this book. Just wrap it up and give it to one of your city friends because you are already living the way you were meant to live. I'm not saying everyone should be working on a farm, but we could all live a lot closer to the way God intends us to live.

We have become jaded. Some of us have never been taught God's ways and we certainly don't see them in the world around us. Every year we get farther and farther away from how God intended us to live. We have become so

[1] Hosea 4:6 (NKJ)

perverted that we now call evil good and good evil. And we can't blame it on others—we *all* do it. Maybe we are not nearly as bad as some who are extremely perverse and evil, but we do it in little things and that's where it all starts, isn't it? I once heard a lady say vehemently to her child, "No! You cannot have any more carrots until you finish your hot dog and chips!" I marveled at how her thinking could have gotten so turned around. I knew the lady well and she was doing what she thought was right, to the best of her ability. But she was ignorant of the right way. We live in a society that wants to push its children to be superhumans instead of teaching them God's ways and how to live in true freedom and simplicity, at peace with God and with their fellowmen.

However, some of us *have* been taught the right way to do things, but we choose not to follow. We have an inner knowledge or voice that shows us the way but we would rather ignore it. "Whether you turn to the right or to the left, your ears will hear a voice behind you saying, 'This is the way; walk in it.'"[2]

Learn to Love Your Body

It is not good to be preoccupied with your body, but it is wise to value the temple God has given you. The Holy Spirit of God dwells in and works through that wonderful body of yours. But how do you treat it? Do you feed it poorly, never allow it to have any exercise, keep it shut away from fresh air and sunshine, fill it with the poisons of unforgiveness and bitterness, never allow it any rest, and then criticize it because it doesn't look good and never does what you want? If that's the case I want to give you your first assignment in this book: STOP THAT!

You must make up your mind to have respect, love, and appreciation for the body God gave you, no matter what shape it is in at this moment. Begin to say to God, as David did, "I praise you because I am fearfully and wonderfully made."[3] Give your body to the Lord as "a living sacrifice,

[2]Isaiah 30:21 (NIV)
[3]Psalm 139:14 (NIV)

holy and pleasing to God."[4]

Your body is a tool of ministry. Do you think you can serve the Lord better in sickness than you can in health? Do you want to serve Him for a couple of decent years, or would you rather have ten, twenty, or thirty more great ones? Our physical condition can influence our spiritual lives far more than we often realize. If we are disciplined in the care of our physical bodies, we are far more likely to be disciplined in our spiritual lives, too.

I don't care how much money Aunt Mildred left you or how good your health insurance is, you cannot afford to be sick. No one can. Sickness detracts from our relationships and service far more than we imagine. God designed the body to be self-repairing and self-healing if we treat it properly. For those of you, like me, who were not healthy to begin with and did not have the advantage of good nutrition and knowledge of God's ways, there is wonderful news. The wonderful news is that the body can be rebuilt in a matter of months. The Seven Steps to Greater Health are a guide to show you how to do it.

Seven Steps to Greater Health

The Seven Steps to Greater Health are based on this Scripture: "For the life of the flesh is in the blood."[5] Now this has a deep spiritual meaning, referring ultimately to the atoning blood of Jesus. But as all Scripture has practical as well as spiritual application, for the purposes of this book we will consider the physical meaning. Remember, God did not just leave us down here to fend for ourselves. He made provisions for the spirit *and* for the flesh.

If the key to life is in the blood, it stands to reason that keeping our bloodstream pure, clean, and healthy is of utmost importance. It doesn't matter how many germs surround you, if the bloodstream is clean, disease cannot breed there. Each of the seven steps contributes to a clean, healthy bloodstream and a system that functions perfectly

[4] Romans 12:1 (NIV)
[5] Leviticus 17:11 (NKJ)

in all areas. The Seven Steps to Greater Health are: (1) peaceful living, (2) pure food, (3) proper exercise, (4) plenty of water, (5) prayer and fasting, (6) fresh air and sunshine, and (7) perfect rest.

Does this sound simple? Well, you're right, the steps *are* simple. God's ways are always beautifully simple. It is *we* who make everything complex. God's ways are perfectly balanced. Man, left to himself, knows no balance. So, although the Seven Steps to Greater Health sound simple, by doing a couple of them to the extreme or by ignoring even one of them, you can make problems for yourself. The key is *balance*. "The man who fears the Lord will avoid all extremes."[6]

The steps are interrelated and interdependent. You can't properly follow one without observing all the others. They are in order from one to seven for good reason. Peaceful living, the first step, is the fountainhead from which all health flows. Perfect rest, the last step, occurs naturally after all the others are in place. Between steps one and seven there is a natural progression with each step preparing the way for the other. Remember: EACH STEP IS DEPENDENT ON THE OTHER SIX—you don't wait until you've mastered step one to move on to step two. You must take a step at a time in each of the seven categories, always checking to see that you're maintaining a balance.

The Seven Steps to Greater Health are a consistent, reliable, preventative way of living that promotes good health. They are intended to add quality and years to your life. We cannot escape death, but we don't have to live in misery all the days of our lives here. All of the seven steps are requirements, not options. They are the minimum requirements for good health.

[6] Ecclesiastes 7:18 (NIV)

Words of Truth

"As for God, His way is perfect."
Psalm 18:30 (NIV)

"You have made known to me the path of life."
Psalm 16:11 (NIV)

"He will teach us His ways, so that we may
walk in His paths."
Isaiah 2:3 (NIV)

"Then you will know the truth, and the
truth will set you free."
John 8:32 (NIV)

"There is a way that seems right to a man
but in the end it leads to death."
Proverbs 16:25 (NIV)

"The fear of the Lord is the beginning of wisdom."
Psalm 111:10 (NKJ)

"The law of the Lord is perfect, reviving the soul."
Psalm 19:7 (NIV)

CHAPTER 1

Step One: Peaceful Living

I know I run a great risk putting a chapter title like this at the beginning of a health book. For one thing, it might cause some of you to put the book down saying, "What does this have to do with health?" Others may be inclined to skip this chapter and go right to the sections on diet and exercise. But because this is a *total* health handbook, I can't begin with anything less than the most important step, the step of securing a consistently peaceful and relatively stress-free life. Without a certain level of peace in one's life, all the exercises and diets in the world aren't going to mean a thing.

I have heard many doctors say that up to ninety-five percent of all illness is related to stress. And even if the illness is not caused by stress, it most certainly is made worse by it — we've all seen people become ill after severe stress, like a death in the family or a divorce.

Margaret, a devoted mother of three closely-spaced children, fell apart when all three of them left home within a short time. Although the children left for very positive reasons, her identity had been threatened and the "empty nest" syndrome hit her hard. She contracted cancer very soon after that, and did not survive.

Jack's forced retirement brought about such great stress that very soon afterward his good health gave way to heart trouble. Having always been a busy, productive, needed person, he began to feel that he was useless and that his life was over. He acted quickly to sell his home and move to a small farm where he could work outside in his vegetable garden and raise a few animals as a service to other farmers. He is now useful, productive, and active. He is also, now, in good health.

The difference between Margaret and Jack is that Jack recognized the signs of stress and was able to do something about it.

Two Kinds of Stress

Stress is the response of your mind, emotions, and body to whatever demands are being made upon you. The crucial part, the part we always forget, is that it's not so much *what* happens to you that determines the effect of stress upon your body, but the way you respond to it. We all have days when something causes us to get angry and depressed, and other days when the same thing might not affect us at all. It all depends on whether we are prepared for the stress. Sometimes it's not a major event that causes stress, but rather a whole bunch of little things added together that are more than we can take.

There are two kinds of stress, positive and negative. Positive stress is happy, good, desirable, controllable, easy to cope with, pleasantly resolvable, and exciting: for example, getting that big work project you've always wanted to do, finding out that the loan for your dream house came through, or coming home to your favorite friends and relatives shouting "Surprise!" as you walk in the door. All of these situations produce happy stress, but it is stress nonetheless, and your body, mind, and emotions have to be kept strong to withstand it.

In contrast, negative stress is sad, maddening, disturbing, uncontrollable, unresolvable, and depressing: for example, serious matters like death and divorce or minor incidents like an argument with your husband, burning your hand on the stove, or getting a traffic ticket. Each of these situations seems out of control. Negative stress takes the greatest toll on the body.

People who cope well with day-to-day negative stress have some kind of outlet or source of inner strength. They don't absorb the stress into themselves. This is because they take charge of daily decisions about what they will allow into their lives and what they will not. They move with a confidence and a knowledge of who they are and who the Lord made them to be. Negative situations may sometimes be out of our control, but our response to them is not. Our response to them is a decision we make. People who absorb the stress and allow themselves to be victimized by situations are the ones who get ulcers.

One good example of allowing negative stress to take control and choosing to be a victim was recently illustrated in my own home. A woman and her two-year-old son came to live with our family. My six-year-old son and two-year-old daughter are very good children who have learned the basic rules of the household — such rules as: Do not write on the wallpaper. Do not upset the potted plants. Do not paint the rug with Mommy's lipstick. Do not flush your "blanky" down the toilet. Now these rules have always seemed basic to me and not unreasonable. However, the visiting mother did not believe in discipline and regularly allowed her child to do all of these things. After about the third week of washing walls, cleaning carpets, vacuuming up potting soil, and calling the plumber, I began to have a deep knot of resentment growing in my stomach. I would go to sleep angry and wake up mad. The stress of it was affecting the rest of the family, too.

Suddenly I realized what I was doing. I was becoming the "poor little victim" by allowing a stressful situation to control me. I was being "Mr. Nice Guy" so everyone would like me. Jesus was never "Mr. Nice Guy" trying to make everyone like him. No, He spoke the truth and did what was right.

So I asked myself, "What is the truth about this situation?" The truth was that the rules in our house ensure everyone's peace and well-being and that, as heads of the household, it is up to my husband and me to see that the rules are enforced.

I went to the woman and apologized for not having told her the rules when she first arrived. It is a mistake to take for granted someone else's knowledge of your household rules. I told her kindly that either she would have to enforce the rules with her son or else we would. She still couldn't bring herself to discipline her child. So from then on, when her son wrote on the walls or rubbed lipstick into the carpet, he got a slap from either me or my husband. It was only a matter of two days and six spankings before the little boy began to see the wisdom of doing things our way. Our home became peaceful once again, the knot in my stomach left, and even the mother seemed relieved. Because I forgot the truth of who I was and what was right, I let myself and my whole family suffer for a month before I did anything about it.

What I learned from this experience is: It is *not* a sin to have rules to live by. It is *not* a sin to correct a child. It *is* a sin to have resentment. It *is* a sin to go to bed with anger. It *is* a sin to be "Mr. Nice Guy," trying to make everyone like you instead of doing what is right. It *is* a sin to invite people into your home and then resent them because they break rules you never told them about. It *is* a sin to try to control other people by having a big list of expectations for them to live up to and then being angry or disappointed when they can't. It *is* a sin to let your body get sick by not controlling the stress around you as much as you possibly can.

We can't control all stress, but we can control how we *react* to it, and we can strengthen our bodies to cope with it.

Sources of Stress

Stress comes from four main sources:

1. *Environment*. Just living in a city can be stressful. Too much noise and pollution, too many people, heavy traffic, competition, isolation, and transience all add up to take their toll on your body and mind. Also, the type of people you live with or near may be positive and uplifting, or negative and upsetting.

2. *Poor diet*. There are foods that are extremely stress producing: Coffee, tea, white sugar, white flour, salt, and highly processed foods with chemical additives, to name a few. I will go into more detail on this subject in the next chapter.

3. *Lack of exercise*. Physical exercise minimizes whatever stress you may have, so a lack of exercise can cause even small amounts of stress to seem monumental.

4. *Your attitude*. We have already said that it is not so much what is happening to you, but your reaction to it that makes the difference. We do so much to torture ourselves with doubt, guilt, worry, and fear, that, in many instances, more damage is done by just thinking about something happening than would be done if the thing actually happened.

Signs of Stress

Every person has their own individual level of tolerance for stress. Something that affects you strongly might be hardly noticed by another. Because of the many changes in body chemistry that happen as a result of prolonged stress, the debilitating physical *and* emotional diseases that result are also highly individual. What produces high blood pressure in one may cause cancer in another. Sometimes stress creeps up on us. We think we are coping well so we don't see the signs. It's important to be aware of the signals of stress in ourselves and in those around us. Some signs of difficulty in coping with stress are tenseness, irritability, depression, the appearance of being in another world, constant fatigue, forgetfulness, low tolerance of frustration, lack of patience, loss of appetite, sleeplessness, frequent headaches, sudden crying over minor things, allergic reactions, constipation, muscular aches and pains, and skin ailments. There are also more serious signs such as high blood pressure, hypertension, premature aging, colitis, ulcers, glandular problems, immune-system breakdown, heart disease, and cancer.

Everything we do produces stress, but when it becomes excessive and more than our bodies can take, then we have problems. Remember that the ultimate reaction to stress is death. We need to recognize stress in our lives before it gets serious and take specific steps to alleviate it.

You may follow all of the other Seven Steps to Greater

Health—including eating right and exercising regularly —but if you do not cope properly with stress, you can end up with serious illness. This is why this first step is crucial.

Two Choices

As I see it there are two alternative ways to deal with stress: do something to change the situation, or learn to "be content whatever the circumstances"[1] and fortify yourself physically, mentally, and spiritually to survive it.

There are many stressful situations that we *can* do something about. For example, if you are living right next to the freeway or airport and the excessive noise is weakening and depleting you, consider moving to more peaceful surroundings. I've known people who moved to the ocean because they loved it so much, but after a few years the noise of crashing waves became so irritating that they had to move inland a few blocks, where they could enjoy the view and have silence at the same time.

If your schedule is stressful, consider taking a time-management course or read a book on the subject and get organized.

If you are a perfectionist, everything that isn't perfect will cause stress in your life.

If you are up against a stressful relationship (let's face it, it's people that most often cause our stress) and you don't see the other person rushing out to take a self-improvement course, take it to God and say, "Okay God, what could you change in *me* that would make this relationship better?" Painful? Yes! Dying to ourselves is always painful. Especially when you are convinced that the other person needs more changing than you. But this kind of pain leads to *life*. The other alternative is just as miserable, and its ultimate end is in disease and agonizing *death*.

So check out your stress sources. Make a list of them. See if there is anything that can be changed to alleviate the problem and then take steps immediately to do just that. If you can't change the situation, do some thinking and maybe some reading about how you can fortify yourself mentally and emotionally to survive the stress in your life.

[1] Philippians 4:11 (NIV)

It's Who You Know

In my own search for peace, I went into Eastern-style mysticism, occult practices, science of this, science of that, positive thinking, self-hypnosis, astrology, numerology, and transcendental meditation. In case you're considering any of these, let me save you the trouble. THEY DON'T WORK! They have great appeal and some of them appear to help temporarily, but they have no lasting value and they are ultimately dangerous. In all of these, the emphasis is on what you *do* (or *don't* do, in some cases). But I have learned that when it comes to peace, both now and eternally, it's who you know that counts. The only true peace you will ever have will come from having a right relationship with God through His Son Jesus Christ, and being filled with His Holy Spirit. All others are fakes! The indwelling Holy Spirit of God produces peace from the inside out like nothing else can. Peace, health, and beauty begin there. You must have a deep, committed, loving walk with God in order to have health in every area of your life.

Early Will I Seek Thee

It's hard to talk to someone you don't know. But it's also hard to get to know people if you don't talk to them. You know how it is with friends: you don't talk as intimately when there are twenty other people listening as you do when it's just the two of you. The same is true of talking with God. You need to have daily time with Him alone — *you* devoted to *Him*. That's how you get to know Him. It's not the same as praying at church, or with your family, or in a prayer group. These are all good, but they can never take the place of your own personal daily communication with God.

Prayer is a means of contacting God and opening up to His purposes for us. The more time you spend with God alone in quiet solitude, the better you will hear His voice guiding and directing you in times of busyness and noise. Doing this on a daily basis will give you a supernatural storehouse of strength and peace that you can draw on throughout the day. That's how you can remain calm when everything around you is chaotic.

Prayer *does* work. Your prayers are *always* heard and they *always* have an effect. Things are set in motion because of them. I've heard people say, "If God knows everything, then He knows what I need and I don't need to ask Him." But God has given us freedom of choice to make our own decisions. It is up to us to take the first step, and then He meets us where we are. He says we don't have to worry about things but we *do* need to ask.

David said, "My voice You shall hear in the morning, O Lord"[2] and "Early will I seek you."[3] Jesus also got up before dawn and went to a solitary place to pray. If we pass up the chance to seek God in prayer early in the morning we will sometimes end up ineffectually grabbing for the time throughout the rest of the day. I've heard it said that we should get close to God before we get close to others. How true! Praying brings wisdom, peace, and a strong mind. Rushing out in the morning having spent little or no time in prayer with the Lord puts us at a definite disadvantage. If you take the time to communicate with the "Control Tower" before you take off on your day, the chances of your life getting out of control are minimized.

For most people, time alone with God is not a spontaneous happening that occurs naturally every day. It is something that has to be planned. If you have to write it down in your date book, do it! Even if it's only for fifteen minutes at first. You must make time for prayer just like you do any other important happening in your life. Other people get to assuming that your time alone with God is not so important and that "surely you can forget it for today," but if you have it written in your date book you can say, "I'm sorry, I have an appointment at half-past seven. Can you come at eight instead?" If you can't pray in the morning, do it when you can. But make it a priority.

You need a quiet place where you won't be interrupted: no television, phone, books, magazines, friends, or family — just you and God. If kneeling beside your bathtub is the only alternative, then do it. God looks on your heart, not

[2] Psalm 5:3 (NKJ)
[3] Psalm 63:1 (NKJ)

your surroundings. If the only time you can find is after the entire world is in bed, or before they get up, then that's the time for you. If you don't find the time, part of your life will just ebb away day after day, and you will slowly erode until you become like a hollow egg shell that cracks under the slightest pressure.

When you go to pray, take your Bible, a notebook, and a pencil. Sometimes God starts telling you many things, and it's good to write them down so you won't forget what you really heard. Also, if the Lord quickens a Scripture for you, or if you are reminded of something you need to jot down, you don't want to have to leave your place of prayer to get a pencil. The last time I did that, I discovered the dog had chewed up a newspaper which I then picked up to throw in the trash, only to realize that the trash needed to be taken out for pickup that morning. On the way out, the phone rang. I answered it and was detained for fifteen minutes, at which point the baby woke up and wanted to be fed. Goodbye prayer time, the race was on. So pick a quiet place and take steps to ensure an uninterrupted time.

Come before the Lord and empty yourself of any worries or concerns. Place everything that you are feeling before the throne of God. Tell Him your hopes, your failures, your disappointments, your secrets. Sometimes total release from all those things can happen right then. Remember that God knows you well and accepts you the way you are. Talk to Him like a close friend or confidant, but don't forget to give Him a chance to answer. Set before Him *everything* in your day and ask Him to bless it. Whatever you give to God is multiplied at least tenfold. This includes time, too. You may devote only fifteen or twenty minutes to God one morning, but you will find that when you give Him your day like that, He helps you to get everything done that you needed to get done. And you've done it in a quiet, orderly, stress-free, and peaceful way. The discipline of spending time alone with God actually enables you to live a more active life. If you are living weakly and feebly, perhaps you are praying weakly and feebly.

Don't forget to pray for all the people you live with (children, husband, roommate, etc.). Your peace depends on

God working in their lives, too.

There will be days when you feel nothing, as though your prayer is accomplishing nothing and you're not getting through. But this is not true. There are seasons like that, so do not be discouraged. Something is *always* being accomplished. Prayer time is calming and relieves stress. It heads off problems before they arise. Time alone with God is vital to your health. Do not neglect it.

Keep 'Fessed Up

Don't have a hidden life and don't keep secrets from God. You must have an absolutely honest relationship with Him or else you're "playing church." So put everything on the line before Him each day. In other words, KEEP 'FESSED UP! Walk out of your prayer closet clean before the Lord. Don't let the devil chain you down with guilt about something when you could easily bring it to God and be free. You can't be compromising or deceptive, especially about yourself and what is in your heart.

"Search me O God and know my heart. See if there is any offensive way in me."[4] If you don't do a daily cleansing, you will end up needing major surgery. Remember, God doesn't have laws for Himself—they're for *us*. Confession is not for *Him*. He already knows the truth. It's for *you!* Think of it this way: The devil wants to shoot you full of poison darts. When you obey the Lord, the darts can't penetrate because you're under His protective covering. When you disobey and don't make it right with God, you've gotten out from under the covering. So when you do something wrong and don't confess it, the devil shoots a dart of guilt in that unprotected area. Get enough darts and you will hardly be able to walk around because you're carrying such a load. It doesn't matter how small the transgression, do not carry around a burden of guilt about it. It's bad for your health. Don't allow the devil to find small uncovered areas in your emotional makeup through which he can shoot a poison dart. When our hearts don't condemn us and the devil can't, then we can have peace.

[4] Psalm 139:23-24 (NIV)

Put On a Garment of Praise

It's very popular right now to have your "colors done" by an expert who shows you what shades are best for you personally. It is amazing to see how people "come alive" when wearing clothes in their correct colors: eyes become bright, skin tone and hair color are enhanced. But there is one garment of *many* colors that is becoming on everyone. It is the garment of praise. I don't know anyone — male or female — who doesn't look more attractive in a "garment of praise instead of a spirit of despair."[5] Praising God invites His presence into our lives and His presence comes to transform us and our circumstances. So if you want more of the Spirit of the Lord in your life, give more of yourself to praise and worship. I once heard worship aptly described as "responding to His love with our love."

Praising God takes the pressure off because it allows Him to breathe life through you and your abilities rather than you trying to do everything yourself. It's *okay* to lose confidence in yourself and your abilities, for then you develop confidence in the Lord's ability to sustain you. So, if you are ever feeling down about what you believe is your lack of talent or gifts, take it to the Lord and begin to worship Him. He will give you all the ability you need and lift your spirit at the same time.

Your attitude toward life will be either one of thankfulness or one of ingratitude. It takes just as much effort to find reasons to be thankful each day as it does to find things to be mad about. So you have a choice to make every morning when you first get up. Will you get up thinking, "Here we go with another lousy day, it's raining, the kids are going to drive me crazy, my husband didn't fix the screen, I'm sure he didn't hear a word I said, nobody appreciates me, what's the use." And as your husband is leaving for work he says, "Goodby, honey, have a good day," at which point you scream at him, "Don't tell me what to do!" The tone of your day is set.

How much more pleasant it would be to get up and say, "This is the day the Lord has made;" I *will* "rejoice and be

[5] Isaiah 61:3 (NIV)

glad in it." [6] And then begin to praise Him for who He is and what He has done. Thank Him for walking with you this day. Thank Him for specific things, large and small, that have happened to you recently: for example, "Thank you Lord for that parking place right in front of the cleaners when I was running late. Thank you for that intimate conversation with my mother. Thank you for protecting me when the cement truck ran the red light. Thank you, God, that Matthew has improved in his schoolwork. Thank you, Father, that I slept well last night." Once you get started being thankful, it's hard to stop. Suddenly you find yourself singing in the shower, smiling at your husband, showing patience to your children, answering the phone with a cheerful voice, and moving through the day with a minimum of stress. And all because you made one decision at the beginning of the day: you chose life instead of death.

When you feel your life getting out of control, or a bad attitude creeping in, begin to praise God. If you're so far down you can't think of anything to be thankful for, at least be grateful you've got a mind and you're still breathing. Start somewhere! God wants us to walk in a spirit of worship, to live in a stance of praise. It's not just a daily occurrence, it's a way of life.

It is very unhealthy to be thinking of ourselves all the time. Focusing inward too much leads to mental problems. Mental hospitals are full of people who do just that. Constantly looking at yourself and asking, "How am I doing? How am I measuring up?" does not bring health. The "me generation" came out with wonderful bodies and very disturbed minds and emotions. There must be a balance between healthy concern for making sure that your body, mind, and spirit are fed adequately, and neurotic *overconcern* with your *self*, which actually produces stress. Focusing everything outward to God is a wonderful, positive way to bring about mental health. The perfect antidote to too much self is praise. Get out of yourself and focus on God. Even the stance that some take of praising God with uplifted hands suggests that you can't hang on to yourself or anything of the world when you let go and lift

[6] Psalm 118:24 (NIV)

your hands to heaven.

Every day is a day of new beginnings. "Behold, I make all things new."[7] His compassions never fail. They are new every morning."[8] Every day you can be excited, joyful, jubilant, full of strength, uplifted, positive, and beautiful when you begin with an attitude of praise for a loving Father. It is one of the most health-building things you can do for every area of your life and being.

How Are You Feeding Your Mind?

What kind of magazines and books are you reading? Are they educational, informative, encouraging? Do you feel like you're a better person after you've read them, or do you feel tired, depressed, dull, and a touch guilty? What about the music that fills your life through the stereo and radio? Is it uplifting and edifying, or is there a spirit of selfishness, greed, unrest, lust, or violence behind it? What about the movies and television programs you watch? Does your television just blare continually all day long, providing a dull background of mindlessness for your life? Is there so much noise from all these things that you wouldn't hear "the still small voice" of God even if He were yelling at you?

In his book *How To Have Good Health* Dr. E. Ted Chandler says that people who watch television more than four hours each day are "more fearful, anxious, and mistrustful than those viewing less than two hours per day." I found this to be true when I was pregnant with my second child. Because I was experiencing a great deal of morning sickness I would let my four-year-old sit in front of the television for hours at a time—something I never let him do normally. He began to have nightmares regularly but I thought it was probably anxiety over how a new sibling would usurp his position as the baby of the family. When I began to feel better and the television was turned off in favor of playing with his toys, the nightmares stopped. I was thankful for the "television babysitter" that I had had during that time, but I became well aware of the damage it could do if it were to become a way of life instead

[7] Revelation 21:5 (NKJ)
[8] Lamentations 3:22-23 (NIV)

of just a temporary measure. Research has shown that too much television reduces a child's ability to think for himself and dulls his mind to such an extent that it affects his work in school. Children who watch more than three hours of television each day seem to do less well in school than those who watch for a shorter time.

Watching television too much, or watching poor-quality programs, is just as destructive for adults as it is for children. There are some excellent programs on television that are informative, uplifting, inspiring, enriching, and fun without being offensive or stupid. Be specific about what you're watching and why. *Do not* be victimized by the television set allowing whatever comes on to come on. Be especially cautious of programs that leave you nostalgic, longing for the "good old days," dissatisfied with your life, depressed with yourself, fantasizing about life with a new husband, a better house, or a meaningful relationship with your best friend's goldfish. Turn off such programs immediately and never let them become a part of your life again. Anything that is of the Lord will never make you feel that way.

Always remember that whatever goes into your mind stays there—you have it filed in your memory forever, and although you may forget it for a time, it is still a part of you. So be careful how you feed your mind because that's what will feed your soul, just as what goes into your stomach will feed your body.

This brings me to the next crucial step in the area of obtaining peace, that is, daily feeding on the Word of God. Reading the Bible is one of the keys to emotional, physical, and spiritual health. God has given us answers to everything in His Word.

Allow me to dispel a myth I often hear. That is that the Bible was written nearly three thousand years ago and is not applicable for today. This is not true! God is a God who "changes not" and He has given us answers for *everything* in His Word. "I am the Lord, I do not change." [9] His Word is physical and practical as well as spiritual and eternal. He

[9] Malachi 3:6 (NKJ)

has included in it everything we need to know for day-to-day living as well as what we need for eternity. Let me repeat: THE BIBLE IS FOR TODAY, IT IS NOT OUT-DATED. "The grass withers, the flower fades, but the Word of our God shall stand forever." [10]

What could be outdated, however, are certain translations. If you have a translation of the Bible that you can't get into and understand, then you have the wrong translation for you. Buy a translation that is easy for you to read and understand. If the King James Version leaves you baffled and frustrated, do not hesitate to get a New International Version or a Living Bible. I know that most Bible scholars and pastors do not prepare their sermons from either of these translations, but I'm not interested in you preparing a sermon, I'm interested in you getting fed by the Truth. If your translation doesn't communicate, find one that does.

Put your own eyes in contact with God's Word. Commit to memory the verses that have special meaning and life for you. Speak the Word of God out loud every day. Don't depend on your pastor, or your minister, or your priest to do it for you. There is a certain growth and richness, a certain confidence and assurance, and a certain hope and joy that can only come when you let the Holy Spirit of God make the Scriptures come alive for you. That's why you cannot read the Bible through once and say, "Okay, I've finished that book. What's next?" The Bible is a book to be read and read again, and each time God will speak to you in a fresh, new way. Every day you will receive from it something different from what you received the day before. That's why the Bible you read today won't be the Bible you'll read next year or five years from now. You may not always realize it, but in the Lord you are always growing. And what helps you to grow and makes you strong and healthy is feeding on the Word of God daily. If you need to write this into your schedule, then do it. It is a step that's more important than you might think.

[10] Isaiah 40:8 (NKJ)

A Time to Laugh, A Time to Cry

You know that old phrase "worried sick"? Well, it's not just an expression — you can worry yourself right into an illness. Doctors have discovered that the opposite is true also. You can laugh your way to health. Laughter normalizes blood pressure, increases the flow of oxygen to the brain and greatly reduces the effects of stress. It is a wonderful quality to be able to find humor in a situation or to be able to laugh at yourself. Because the body is directly affected by what happens in the mind, a life with an abundance of laughter and joy promotes good health. Is there enough laughter in your life? "A cheerful heart is good medicine, but a crushed spirit dries up the bones,"[11] and "a cheerful heart has a continuous feast."[12]

Crying is also good for you sometimes. And, interestingly enough, it has some of the same physical benefits as laughter. Researchers say that sick people cry less than healthy people and that people with stress-related problems are more likely than healthy people to view crying as a sign of weakness or lack of control. They've discovered that there are certain elements contained in emotionally induced tears that are not present in tears that are artificially induced (as, for example, by peeling an onion). Could it be that these elements are a result of stress buildup and can only be released by crying? A free flow of tears appears to be a wonderfully healthy, natural release from stress. In fact, restricting your tears can be detrimental to your health. So if you feel led to tears for *any* reason, go ahead and cry — and this goes for you men, too! Okay, if you don't want to cry in front of your boss when the promotion doesn't come through or be reduced to sobs in public when the Dodgers lose, then go into the privacy of your office, bathroom, car, closet, pantry, garage, or tree house. Why be the one to have a heart attack or cancer at age forty-five just because of some false image of you that society invents. Jesus cried, and there has never been a more perfect man.

My son, Christopher, would never cry in front of his father. He could cry his heart out to me, but if his father

[11] Proverbs 17:22 (NIV)
[12] Proverbs 15:15 (NIV)

walked in the room, Christopher would immediately pull himself together. That concerned me, so I asked a friend and counselor about it. She said, "It's probably because he has never seen his dad cry." Michael and I thought about the situation and realized that this was true. While my husband is freer than most men in allowing himself to cry in front of me, he never cried in front of our son. I, on the other hand, am a pretty prolific cryer and have always cried freely in front of just about anybody. We took steps to change the situation and were totally amazed at a change in Christopher from the "military-school syndrome" to being totally open about crying in front of his dad. That says a lot for living a full life in terms of our emotions, doesn't it? We must let them come out rather than denying or supressing them. Crying, even though it is most often a reaction to something negative, is a positive, healthy reaction that we should allow ourselves more often.

Out of the Overflow of the Heart

It says in the Bible that when we see God face to face we will have to give account for every careless word that we have spoken. What a frightening thought. But I believe that we also have to *pay* for our careless words here and now. There is in the tongue the power of life and death. What you say can either bring life to you and your situation, or it can bring death.

"Pleasant words are a honeycomb, sweet to the soul and healing to the bones." [13] "The mouth of the righteous is a fountain of life" [14] and "a deceitful tongue crushes the spirit." [15] To live truly in peace, you must watch what comes out of your mouth. The only way to control that is to go to the source of all expression, that is, to the heart. "For out of the overflow of the heart the mouth speaks. The good man brings good things out of the good stored up in him, and the evil man brings evil things out of the evil stored up in him." [16]

[13] Proverbs 16:24 (NIV)
[14] Proverbs 10:11 (NIV)
[15] Proverbs 15:4 (NIV)
[16] Matthew 12:34-35 (NIV)

Have you ever said things to your children, your husband, a friend, or a stranger that you wish you hadn't said? So have I. You can say you didn't mean it and that you're sorry, but still the words have been spoken. God created the world by speaking the Word. Because we are made in His image, He gives us creative power to speak *our* worlds into existence, too. We can have a world of disharmony, strife, suspicion, and hatred just by speaking a few words of death into a situation.

If you say to your son, "You dummy, you're never going to amount to anything," are you speaking life into the boy, into yourself, or into your relationship with him, or are you speaking something that kills? Again, we have to make a choice for life or for death. When words are blurted out of our mouths that we will later regret, this is a sign of negative heart overflow. When this happens, check what is going on inside of you. Are you holding on to any anger, bitterness, or resentment? If you are, it should be confessed to the Lord immediately and then, if you feel the need, talk to a friend about it.

Keeping anger inside is killing. Nowhere in the Bible does it say you should never get angry, but it does say, "In your anger do not sin. Do not let the sun go down while you are still angry, and do not give the devil a foothold." [17] This means that when you are angry you should deal with it immediately. Confront it, take it to God, and take it to the person who caused the anger. If you keep negative emotions in they will come out in your body. Always be caught up on your feelings so they won't flow out of your mouth with the overflow of your heart.

Unforgiveness is one of the most devastating of all negative emotions. It's a slow and painful killer; it grows like a cancer. In fact, unforgiveness and serious illness may be more closely related than we care to realize. Suppose someone did something terrible to you. Would you say to yourself, "I'll never forgive him for this"? This attitude is guaranteed to make you sick and it doesn't matter whether your unforgiveness is warranted. It's God's job to judge and sentence because He's the only one who knows the whole

[17] Ephesians 4:26-27 (NIV)

story. We can never have enough facts to judge others, no matter how well we feel we know them. Remember that forgiving someone doesn't make them right, it makes *you free*. Don't shorten your life, or greatly impair the quality of it, by giving in to unforgiveness. Deal with it on a daily basis. Ask yourself, "Which would I rather have: forgiveness and peace or unforgiveness and cancer?" It helps you to make a decision.

Damaged Emotions

Some of us have habits of thinking that were established in a troubled or traumatic childhood. We're all grown-up and we find we're unable to love ourselves and don't know how to love others. Our emotions have been damaged and we're left with deep-seated feelings of inferiority.

Everybody has some feelings of inferiority, but some people are truly paralyzed by them. God never intended us to be scarred like that. He created us to be whole in every way and I'm here to tell you that you still can be. This is not the book for me to go into detail about my own personal victory over this problem, but let me say simply that God has healed my broken, wounded inner self and He will heal you, too, because God has no favorites. He responds to all people who seek Him. However, I did not do it on my own and it did not happen overnight. I had a great church, with a wonderful pastor and excellent counselors. They stayed with me until I was free. If you're severely injured, you need help from *good Christian counselors, pastors,* and *psychologists*. I'll tell you right now that the world doesn't have the answers. I thank God for the world's psychologists and psychiatrists who help us to understand and cope with this problem, but there is only one Deliverer—His name is Jesus. That's why it is crucial to seek the help of counselors who know *the* Counselor. Do not give up until you are free from the stress of crippling emotions.

Be Who You Were Created To Be

I passed an old man on the street the other day who was filthy, ragged, stooped, listless, and repulsive. He was pushing a shopping cart full of dirty, smelly old rags, and I

knew they were all his worldly belongings. He was one of
the "street bums" who don't have homes but live outdoors
and carry everything they own around with them. He asked
me for a quarter. I said "Sir, I don't have a quarter but I do
have a twenty-dollar bill I would like to give you." His
weather-worn old hands shook as he took the bill and
kissed it. With tears in his eyes he smiled and said, "Oh,
thank you, miss, thank you!" and began to walk off. I would
like to be able to tell you that I took the man home; gave
him a warm bath, a clean bed, and a good job; and
introduced him to Jesus, but that didn't happen. I did,
however, take him home with me in my heart, and as I
prayed for him I began to feel the deep pain that I've felt so
many times before when I've seen people who have never
realized what the Lord made them to be. The grief I felt
must be a tiny fraction of what the Father feels when He
sees a son or daughter whose life has become a twisted,
distorted, perverted remnant of what it was originally
intended to be. God never created that old man to be like
that. Inside him, just as inside all of us, God placed specific,
purposeful, magnificent gifts, but that old street bum never
found out who He is in the Lord. And I thought how true
that is of so many of us. We may even know the Lord, but
we never take the time or effort to find out who we are made
to be. We walk around with the emotional and spiritual
equivalents of filthy rags and beg for quarters when He
wants to give us His Kingdom. How many of us have
allowed a worldly mind instead of the mind of Christ to
influence our choices in life?

Do you know that one tremendous source of constant
stress is working at a job that you don't like? I'm not
talking about a temporary job to help you pass from one
point to another; I'm talking about a lifelong occupation.
There is a debilitating form of constant stress in the world
today and it comes from people being molded into an image
other than God's.

How about you? Do you love what you do? Would you
rather be doing what you're doing than anything else?
Don't get me wrong. I realize that the best job on earth has
times of frustration, boredom, and dirty work. But most of

the time are you happy and excited and eager to do your job? If not, you should check with the Lord right away to see if you're where He wants you to be and are doing what you were created to do best.

Are you a computer programmer when you should have been a farmer, or a doctor when you should have been a musician, or a bank teller when you should be working in a preschool, or an insurance salesman when you should have been a pastor, or an accountant when you should have been a veterinarian? It is important to your health to do work that you love to do. You will always do that best, and you will be free of the frustration and stress that comes with not being what you were created to be.

If you've been called to motherhood, do you love being a mother? If being a mother is all boredom, strain, and unfulfillment you should check to see if you are denying something about yourself. Has God gifted you with painting, decorating, gardening, writing, or some other talent that you are not using? If that's true, may I ask you why? Are you trying to be Supermom instead of being a super mom? If God has gifted you with painting (or the desire to paint), take an art class and set up a place where you can paint while the baby is taking a nap. That doesn't mean you deny your motherhood; it means that along with all the wonderful God-given responsibilities of your life, you don't deny your personhood. Remember, it is *not* a sin to take an art class, but it *is* a sin to sit around hating your life. You will find that your greatest ministry will be in doing what you most enjoy. You will bless others best with that which blesses you.

Gary, our accountant, is very successful at what he does because he loves his work. He gets every bit as excited about dealing with numbers as I do about writing lyrics to a song.

We have a housekeeper named Thelma who loves to putter around the house and keep it clean and pretty. She had left us a couple years ago for a very good-paying job as a saleswoman. She ended up with ulcers and insomnia and came back to work for us, where it is calm and peaceful and there is no pressure. You can tell by her high-quality work and her good attitude that she is happy doing what she is doing.

There is a very special man who works for us frequently. I believe that there isn't a thing that Dennis cannot build or repair. His work is of the highest quality and he is always pleasant to be around.

Our mechanic Peter has a degree in engineering and once accepted a high-paying position in a large company. After a few years he decided that being a mechanic was something he loved more, so he went back to working on cars. His work is so superior that he is now able to set up his own shop.

These people didn't happen into our lives by accident. We chose them because their attitude is wonderful and their work is of the highest quality. That's because they are doing what they were created to do.

You will never find total health or total peace—or total anything—in life if you are working against what you were created to be and do. I'm not talking about the times when the Lord puts you in a place for a while to learn something. I'm talking about you choosing an occupation or lifestyle, not because the Lord directed you to do it or placed a desire in your heart for it, but because of external factors, such as money, glamour, social status, or fulfilling the expectations of your parents or your peers. These worldly enticements can never substitute for finding the high calling that God has placed upon your life.

How do you find out whether the desires of your heart are from God? You lay down those desires before the Lord and be willing to give them up totally if that's what He asks you to do. When I came to the Lord I was working as an actress and a writer. After about a year I laid both of those things before the Lord and said, "Lord I want to be what you want me to be." He took the acting away and He let me keep the writing. The doors to acting closed and the doors to writing opened. A few years later I realized how wrong acting would have been for me. I pursued it for the glamour and the attention and the false feeling of being loved that it gave me. Writing I did because I thoroughly loved and enjoyed it.

Because I love writing so much I do not deny it as a part of myself. I make time for it. Do you know where and when I wrote this book? In the dentist's office, at the hairdresser's, during the baby's nap, on airplane flights, before everyone was up, after everyone was in bed, in the park while the children played, in my car while I waited to pick up my son from school, in the library when I had a spare hour. When you love doing something you can find the time for it. I would love to go away for a couple of months and just write but that is not an option for me and I don't see it being one during the next twenty years. So I work within the structure of my life as the Lord has arranged it. I take pains not to neglect my husband or my kids or my health or my time with God. With the money I've made from writing I can now afford a housekeeper, but for most of my life I didn't have that. When I had my first baby and had to have a writing project completed, I organized a babysitting co-op with two other mothers. I took their children on Monday mornings and they took mine on Wednesdays and Fridays. That entire project was written between nine and noon two days a week. The Lord knew I had little time and He blessed the time I had.

If I can do it, so can *you*. Ask yourself these questions: Do I love what I am doing? Would I be happy doing it even if I weren't being paid? What would I enjoy doing most? Am I in a line of work that causes negative stress? Do I resent what I do? Do I always feel like I can't wait to get away from my work? Is this something God really has called me to do?

We were never meant to live under the stress of feeling useless, bored, and chronically out of place. Check out your work. See whether it causes stress or brings fulfillment. The best work you'll ever do in your life is the work you most enjoy. Be who you were created to be and you'll find out what you were created to do.

Simplify, Simplify, Simplify

Is your life moving too fast? Is there never enough time to do anything well and feel good about it? Are you always rushing? Are your children taking piano lessons, swim-

ming lessons, ballet lessons, guitar lessons, soccer, baseball, football, yo-yo, when they could perhaps do without
some activities and really focus on one or two in such a way
as to get more enjoyment out of them? Are you trying to be
Superwoman? Could you yourself be more selective about
the things you do rather than have forty things going at
once?

Calmness and strength are lost in too much busyness and
rush. "In quietness and trust is your strength." [18] When you
hurry through life there is a wonderful quality of living you
miss altogether. A certain depth of communication with the
Lord is also lost. If your schedule rules out time for a friend
in need, for something unexpected, for periods of solitude
and listening to God, for being alone with each child, for
staying within the speed limit, and for getting away alone
with your husband, you need to reexamine your priorities
and schedule. There may be seasons of busyness, but they
cannot be allowed to become a way of life. The cost is too
great.

If you live in the city, vacations away are vital to your
health. Make sure they offer a complete change of scenery
and something that reverses the rhythm of your normal
pace, such as going to the mountains, the beach, or to a
farm or a ranch. Anything that gets you closer to the world
God created and away from the world man made promotes
peace. It's important to get back to a simpler life to gain
proper perspective.

"But I fear, lest somehow, as the serpent deceived Eve by
his craftiness, so your mind may be corrupted from the
simplicity that is in Christ." [19] In that statement Paul
expressed to the Corinthians his concern that the deceptive
enemy of peace not creep in to rob them of the beauty of the
simple life we are intended to live in the Lord. Beloved one
in Jesus, this is my prayer for you, too. Let the word
SIMPLICITY be always in your mind as you make your
choices each day. Let simplicity guide you through your
decisions and plans. Don't allow your life to get too
complex. If you have too many responsibilities, belongings,

[18] Isaiah 30:15 (NIV)
[19] II Corinthians 11:3 (NKJ)

gadgets, obligations, meetings, payments, clothes, jobs, or phone calls, get rid of some of them. Before you buy anything ask yourself, "Will this make my life simpler or more complex?" Get rid of things you can live without so you can better care for all that you love. Simplicity brings peace.

What Will You Choose?

"For whoever would love life and see good days...must seek peace and pursue it." [20] So you see we can even choose whether to be happy or sad. Isn't that amazing? And all along we thought we were the victims.

Because the mind influences the body we must always make efforts to control it. Fear, worry, depression, anxiety, resentment, and self-pity bring stress that interferes with every process in your body. It depletes your store of energy and actually poisons you. If your mind and emotions suffer, so will your whole body and no amount of exercising and dieting will alleviate it. When you are under stress, everything is thrown off, and you don't eat properly and can't eliminate properly. All this causes nervous exhaustion, which keeps you from sleeping and makes you feel like staying in bed until Jesus comes.

Nobody can avoid stress altogether but you can do many things to minimize it and to soften your reactions to it. Sometimes we are so busy that we fail to notice or to understand stress signals. But if you are faithfully observing all of the Seven Steps to Greater Health, you will be able to handle unavoidable major stress without falling apart. Be aware that when you are under stress your body needs more care than at other times. Stress is relieved by a right relationship with God, eating food the way God made it, physical exercise, drinking plenty of pure water, fasting, getting enough fresh air, sunshine, and rest—in other words, by following *all* of the Seven Steps to Greater Health.

There will always be too many things to do, a house that needs to be cleaned, and people who need you (children will

[20] I Peter 3:10 (NIV)

never have enough of you). Be sure you have something to give them by drawing apart and communicating with the Father, the true source of all peace. Be filled with Him. "The Lord blesses His people with peace." [21] We always have two options in everything we do: we can make choices for life or choices for death. Which will you choose?

[21] Psalm 29:11 (NIV)

Words of Truth

"There is a future for the man of peace."
Psalm 37:37 (NIV)

"A heart at peace gives life to the body."
Proverbs 14:30 (NIV)

"The mind of sinful man is death, but the mind
controlled by the Spirit is life and peace."
Romans 8:6 (NIV)

"A man's own folly ruins his life, yet his heart
rages against the Lord."
Proverbs 19:3 (NIV)

"The fruit of righteousness will be peace; the effect
of righteousness will be quietness
and confidence forever."
Isaiah 32:17 (NIV)

"Great peace have they who love Your law,
and nothing can make them stumble."
Psalm 119:165 (NIV)

"Be anxious for nothing, but in everything by
prayer and supplication, with thanksgiving,
let your requests be made known unto God;
and the peace of God, which surpasses all
understanding, will guard your hearts
and minds through Christ Jesus."
Philippians 4:6-7 (NKJ)

CHAPTER 2

Step Two: Pure Food

Countless books and articles have been published on the subject of nutrition. Nothing else evokes so much interest, debate, and controversy. It appears that no two authorities agree on everything: one says, "high protein," another says, "high carbohydrate," another, "vegetarianism." Others say, "no eggs," "yes, eggs," "no milk," "raw milk only," "honey is good," "honey is bad," "sugar gives you energy," "sugar will kill you," "no salt," "we'll die without salt," "yes, vitamins," "we don't need vitamins," "yes, meat," "no meat!" By the time we count our calories, multiply the proteins, divide by the fats, weigh our portions, reduce our grams, and count the cost of every bite, we are so weary of it all that a "candy bar and soft drink" sounds like a better solution.

And yet we long to know the truth so that we aren't driven all over the grocery store by every food fad that comes along. A simple thing like eating has gotten too complex. Confusing, complex, unbalanced, difficult-to-understand rules were never established by God. They couldn't be, because God's ways are orderly, simple, balanced, and clear. Anything else is not from God. God's ways are also pure and natural. Anything else must have been processed by man.

Originally the choices were simple. You ate what was available in each season. But now you have the choice of any kind of food at any time you want it. And if you have enough money, it can be flown in from halfway around the world and delivered to your house so you'll never even have to leave your television. We are continually surrounded by too much food that is too easily accessible. At the prompting of a television commercial, we can rush to the nearest fast-food store and in a matter of seconds be stuffing ourselves full of a form of food that we were never intended to eat in the first place. Many people have plenty to eat but suffer from malnutrition. They are under-nourished because they don't know what to choose.

I have learned a way of eating that is simple, balanced, and easy to understand, and it has never let me down in the health area. It is a "way of life for eating," not a diet. It is the way to eat whether you need to lose weight, gain weight, stay the same, or get well. It is totally satisfying and you do not have hunger as a way of life. To sum it up in a nutshell it is: EATING PURE FOOD THE WAY GOD MADE IT, or as close as possible to the way He made it.

Processed or Pure

Certain foods destroy health. They fill your body with toxic poisons and somewhere down the road you will have to pay for it. Our foods have been so processed and robbed of life-giving vitamins, minerals, and digestive enzymes, that they are a perversion of what God intended. Man started doing things to these wonderful natural foods God gave us to make them look "more attractive," be "instantly prepared," and "last forever" on the grocery shelf. He stripped the life out of them and added chemical preservatives, artificial flavors and colors, and synthetic vitamins. He changed them into devitalized and sometimes danger-ous foods. We are sick and overweight because we eat more refined food than we do natural pure food.

Only God can create life, and only pure food the way God made it is life giving. Foods that are not natural will always interfere with your body's functions in some way. Natural foods, the way God made them or as close as possible to the way He made them, promote health, strength, endurance, and life. Processed foods promote disease and death.

God designed the best foods for us to sustain life. He gave us fruits, vegetables, grains, nuts, and seeds that have the

perfect balance of vitamins, minerals, and digestive
enzymes. "And God said, 'See I have given you every herb
that yields seed which is on the face of all the earth, and
every tree whose fruit yields seed; to you it shall be for
food.'"[1] Later, after the flood, God said to Noah, "Everything that lives and moves will be food for you,"[2] which
added meat to our diet.

God didn't leave anything out when He made food. He
made it perfect and we can't improve on it. Some companies
claim that their refined foods can build bodies eight ways,
ten ways, or twelve ways. How good is that when natural
food the way God made it can build bodies in as many as
fifty ways?

I've seen people who were sick and feeble grow strong and
healthy by getting their mind off stressful things, com-
muning with God and His creation, and learning to eat food
the way God made it. I saw this first hand when my father
had a severe heart attack at about sixty years of age. There
had been no major signs of illness before that, except that
he had been about forty pounds overweight. After the
attack, the doctor put him on a very strict vegetable diet.
Only fresh raw or steamed vegetables for *every* meal for
what seemed like eternity to my dad but was only about
four months. He looked gravely ill in the hospital, but over
the weeks of recovery and strict diet he became a new
person. He lost all the extra weight, his blue eyes became
bright and clear, his skin became soft, smooth, and healthy
in color. He recovered totally and has just celebrated his
seventy-fifth birthday in good health. I thank God for
doctors who are aware of God's ways. My dad's case was an
extreme condition that called for extreme measures. We
don't need to live that extremely but it proves that natural
foods restore health.

The more you know about the way God made food and
how He intended for you to eat it, the easier it will be for you
to make choices for life instead of for death in the area of
your diet. Remember that God's ways are good, pure,
natural, balanced, and cannot be improved.

[1] Genesis 1:29 (NKJ)
[2] Genesis 9:3 (NIV)

The same is true for the food God made. The more processes it goes through before it gets to your body, the less it will have to offer. When you eat refined, processed, devitalized foods, your body is not nourished and you don't feel satisfied, so you overeat to make up for it. "Let us purify ourselves from everything that contaminates body and spirit, perfecting holiness out of reverence for God." [3] Separating yourself from anything that defiles you is a much higher purpose than catering to your physical appetites. "Everything is permissible — but not everything is beneficial." [4]

Life and Death Are in the Blood

We have sixty trillion cells in our bodies. (I don't know who counted them.) Every cell lives for a limited time before it reproduces itself and dies. Every three months we get a new bloodstream, every eleven months each cell in our body has been renewed, and every two years we get a new bone structure. Do you realize that by eating correctly for approximately two years, you could have a whole new body? I don't mean that you could all of a sudden look like someone else, but you could certainly be a totally new *you*. Isn't that encouraging?

The idea behind good health is to keep your blood clean through proper foods, *plus* exercise, plenty of water, fasting and prayer, fresh air and sunshine, and peaceful, stress-free living. *Eating food the way God made it affects the blood by cleansing it from impurities and by supplying it with all the nutrients necessary to rebuild cells.* The Lord's way of eating will keep your blood clean and healthy, and this will automatically protect you from infection. A dirty bloodstream is the main cause of illness and premature aging. When the bloodstream is pure and alkaline, it will dissolve all poisons and carry them away. Disease cannot live in a clean bloodstream. Disease breeds in a dirty bloodstream.

Keeping the bloodstream clean, and the body healthy, requires personal discipline. *You* must supervise what goes into your stomach. How are you feeding your sixty trillion

[3] II Corinthians 7:1 (NIV)
[4] I Corinthians 10:23 (NIV)

cells? Are they being fed food that has no vitamins, minerals, or digestive enzymes? Are they being fed food that is so devitalized that your body has to spend precious energy just trying to rid itself of poisonous wastes and repair the damage that your food has done?

The human body can take years of punishment before it rebels against being loaded down with foodless foods and the toxic poisons they produce. When the body cannot undo the damage done to it fast enough, the bloodstream becomes clogged and dirty. Then the whole system begins to break down and becomes a breeding ground for disease, which results in premature aging. This does not have to happen. We were created to be alive until we die, not dying the whole time we're alive. You can enjoy good health as a way of life but it will only be found in living the way God intended us to live and eating food the way God intended us to eat it.

Bad Food and Body Breakdown

I have read many articles on how good nutrition can save marriages, reduce crime, empty the mental hospitals, and generally make us better persons. While I don't believe the answer to these problems is diet alone, I am sure that poor nutrition does exacerbate them. A marriage has got to suffer if both partners are chronically fatigued and plagued with aches, pains, constant sickness, and depression, as opposed to being healthy, strong, and clear-minded. There are certain mental disorders that can definitely be relieved by a pure diet, and who knows how many crimes or abuses wouldn't have been committed if the criminal had been feeling strong, clear-minded, and rational, rather than weak and overwhelmed by his life and circumstances. I've heard it said by experts in the field that people carry between five and twenty pounds of toxic poisons and wastes inside of them. Shocking, isn't it? But if all those poisons don't get out, our body breaks down under the stress, we become sick, and personal relationships are affected.

Toxic wastes build up in your body when you eat too many impure, processed, foodless foods and don't give your

body a chance to rest and get rid of them. The body will
naturally try to purify and cleanse itself. If you help it by
providing food the way God made it, exercise, rest, fresh air
and sunshine, plenty of water, regular fasting, and a good
attitude, you will have a clean bloodstream and a healthy
body.

Disease does not come overnight. It builds for a long time.
In *Back to Eden* Jethro Kloss made an interesting point:
"When the minerals and vitamins, which would keep the
body symmetrical, are removed from the food, we grow all
out of shape and proportion, and it makes us subject to all
kinds of diseases." To take the mystery out of being sick,
think of disease as another way of saying "out of balance."
Whenever you feel yourself getting sick, try to figure out
where you got out of balance. Check each of the seven steps
to see if you've neglected any. If you get too far out of
balance you need the help of a professional nutritionist or,
if you have a disease, a medical doctor. You should never
put off going to a medical doctor if you really need one, but
to run to a doctor for every sniffle is unnecessary since God
has given us a way to balance ourselves again.

If you have been suffering from obscure ailments and the
doctor can't find anything wrong with you even though you
know you "feel crummy" most of the time, you might have
an accumulation of poisons and toxic wastes in your
system. Wherever you have a weakness in the body poisons
will settle because weak tissues are unable to eliminate
wastes properly. A weak area will flare up again and again:
the same sinus condition, throat infection, ear infection,
stomach problem, aching shoulder, or just plain "crummy
feeling." This is one of the indications that you have a toxic
buildup. Eating food the way God made it begins to flush
out all the poisons.

Fruits and vegetables are *eliminating* and *cleansing*
foods, and are *alkaline forming. Starches and proteins* are
body builders, and are *acid forming.* You always want a
more alkaline body. A too acidic condition breeds disease.
There must always be a proper balance, but we all tend to
eat not enough of the alkaline-forming eliminative fresh
fruits and vegetables. Poisons move out of the body when

raw or properly cooked fruits and vegetables are eaten. If you've been feeling weak, check to see if you are getting enough of the body purifiers — fresh fruits and vegetables.

I always used to suffer from seasonal colds and flu. But when I eat pure food the way God made it, I do not get these things at all. The same is true for the rest of my family. Because of our human inconsistencies and the fact that a certain amount of impurities creep into everything, we set aside three special times of the year for a week of cleansing. In our family, the cleansing diet begins with a three-day fast (the children don't fast) and then we eat only a wide variety of fresh fruits and vegetables for a few days after that. It cleans out the system and we feel great afterward. We have found that the best times for this are:

1. *January*, after Christmas and New Year's celebrations are over, and we need to make up for our indulgence in the wonderful temptations of the season.

2. *Late spring* (in May is good), to prepare you for the seasonal change to summer. You will be surprised how much more resistance you will have to spring colds and hay fever.

3. *September*, when you're about to change your style of living again, this time from summer to fall. The temperature is about to drop and, as a result, this time has become known as the "cold" season. Don't fall prey to that. Go on a cleansing diet for a week and see if it doesn't help you avoid the traditional fall or winter cold or flu.

A strict diet of fresh fruits and vegetables may not seem fun at first but you'll find that it is a lot more fun than being sick. In the Bible, Daniel was aware of the advantages of this way of eating:

> "Please test your servants for ten days: Give us nothing but vegetables to eat and water to drink. Then compare our appearance with that of the young men who eat the royal food, and treat your servants in accordance with what you see. So he agreed to this and tested them for ten days. At the end of the ten days

they looked healthier and better nourished than any of
the young men who ate the royal food."[5]

If you have a problem eating fruit, stick with vegetables
until your body balances itself. Remember, this is just a
week of cleansing. You're not to stick to this way of eating
all the time, but you must go back to the balance between
building foods and cleansing foods. When you go on a
cleansing diet for a week you may find that you have a
headache, chills, or diarrhea for a few hours, or what seems
like hay fever or a slight cold. Do not be alarmed by this, it
is just poison coming out of the system. It will come and go
quickly, and when it is over you will feel stronger than ever.
Drink plenty of water and pure herb teas to help flush out
the body.

You will find that your whole mental attitude and outlook
will change when you are free from the toxic poisons in
your system. I am convinced that many depressions are
caused by poisons in the body. I have seen many cases
where nothing else in a person's situation changed, but by
eating correctly their outlook and attitude improved. You
will eventually find that you enjoy being well so much that
turning down doughnuts and coffee will be easy. Merely
eating simply and naturally prevents a lot of disease and
pain.

Foods That God Made

Many dietary elements are necessary to produce good
health. When any one element is missing, this weak link
causes the whole body to break down. However, you don't
have to sit with charts and a calculator at each meal to see
if you are getting everything you need. You do not need to
supply every needed element each time you sit down to eat,
or even every day. If you pay attention to this seven-point
list and include all of it *each week* you will do very well and
life will be very simple:

1. *Vegetables and fruits:* Only fresh, not canned, frozen,
   processed in any way. Eaten raw, lightly steamed,
   baked, or stewed. Vegetables and/or fruits must make up

[5] Daniel 1:12-15 (NIV)

fifty percent of every meal. In fact, it is best if you can start every meal with something raw, like fruit for breakfast and vegetables for lunch and dinner. Use a wide variety of each so you are not eating the same thing every day.

2. **Whole grains:** They can comprise twenty-five percent of one meal, or, at the most, twenty-five percent of two meals each day. In other words, if you have a whole-grain toast, muffin, or waffle for breakfast and you know you are going to have a whole-grain rice for dinner, do not have any grain at lunch. And remember, whenever you have grains of any kind, they should not be in greater quantity than twenty-five percent of the meal.

3. **Meat, poultry, and fish:** Select only one of these each day, at whatever meal you prefer. Have the red meats no more than two times a week, poultry two or three times a week, and fish two times a week. Let meat, poultry, or fish be no more than twenty-five percent of the meal. To put it in the simplest terms, let's say, at dinner tonight, for example, fifty percent of the food you eat should be the vegetable salad and the steamed carrots, twenty-five percent the roast chicken, and twenty-five percent the wild rice. If you arrange your portions with this in mind, you will keep a healthful balance of alkaline- and acid-forming foods. Always keep in mind that red meat is digested slowly, so you won't want to eat too much of it too often.

4. **Seeds, nuts, and berries:** These make wonderful "munchies," snacks, and desserts. You can buy nuts and seeds in the shell and hull them yourself for greater nutritional value, or purchase them in packages that say "raw" on the label. Seeds are regenerating and rejuvenating and are rich in protein and minerals. Most nuts that you find in the market are roasted and salted and, as a result, have lost much of their nutritional value and are more difficult to digest. This is especially true of peanut butter. When peanut butter has been processed, overcooked, and salted, it becomes a constipating, difficult-to-digest food. Buy it unprocessed, or eat plain

raw nuts when you can. Excellent choices that are easy
to find are: almonds, walnuts, pecans, chestnuts,
cashews, hazelnuts, and pistachios. All berries make
great desserts and are totally healthful and non-
fattening.

5. *Milk, unprocessed cheese, yogurt, kefir, cottage
cheese, and butter:* Only three or four times a week
for these—not each of them three or four times a week,
but rather three or four times a week you can pick one of
them. Milk and milk products must be taken in modera-
tion. Of course, they should be in the purest form
available. In other words, by buying yogurt that has
been cooked at such a high temperature that the good
bacteria have been killed, with sugar added to sweeten,
artificial flavors added to make you think you're eating
strawberries, and chemicals to make it last forever, you
end up with a food that God never intended you to eat.
Yogurt is easy to make yourself if you can't find a
natural source.

6. *Eggs:* Two or three times a week only, and as fresh as
you can get them. Fertilized eggs have more nutrients,
but are not available everywhere.

7. *Honey:* Honey is the most nutritious natural sweetener
that you can get if you buy it "raw," "unprocessed," and
"unfiltered." Just like anything else, if it has been
cooked and processed the life has been taken out of it.
Throughout the Bible it is mentioned as a wonderful
food to be used with wisdom and balance. Those who
malign honey and say that it is as bad as sugar are
talking about honey that has been processed. Sugar
used now and then is not going to kill you. Sugar every
day will be hazardous to your health. Natural sugar
cane, just like natural salt, has vitamins and minerals
in it, but commercial refining takes all its benefits away
and leaves us with a good-tasting, slow-working poison.
Refined sugar in frequent high doses can cause diabetes,
hypoglycemia, tooth decay, mental problems, learning
disabilities, and vitamin-B shortage. Sugar substitutes
are just as dangerous as sugar. It's only a matter of

time before you are totally saturated with chemical sweeteners and have to pay the price in your health. Honey, on the other hand, is filled with minerals and is an aid to digestion, as well as a help in preventing sore throats, colds, raw nerves, and insomnia. It has wonderful qualities—if you don't overdo it.

This is a very basic list but you will do very well if you abide by it. To help you along, buy a good health-conscious cookbook and use it to get ideas. There is no reason why food the way God made it should ever taste bad. However, there are many things we need to learn about preparing foods properly. A salad, for example, is not just a quarter of a head of lettuce slapped into a bowl with a glob of some orange or white gooey stuff on top. That's the way I have seen it in many restaurants and that is not a salad! A real salad includes different types of green lettuce, like red leaf, romaine, or endive, and some nicely chopped green peppers, carrots, celery, cucumbers, tomatoes, green onions, and avocados. For variety, add shredded beets, raw zucchini, cabbage, spinach leaves, raw broccoli, cauliflower, and different kinds of sprouts. For a dressing use natural unprocessed oil, apple-cider vinegar and/or the juice of a lemon, and some natural seasonings.

Steamed vegetables don't have to be boring, either. Green beans, for example, can be lightly steamed, and placed in a bowl with two or three tablespoons of oil and one whole onion, chopped or sliced. Toss the ingredients together and let them sit in a bowl with a clean dish towel over the top for five to ten minutes. Take the towel off the top and serve them without the onions (or with, if you like raw onions); the onion flavor will have penetrated the beans. Our whole family loves them, including our two-year-old.

When buying or eating food always remember that the more processes a food has to go through before it gets to you, the quicker you should decide against buying and eating it. The more devitalized and processed foods you eliminate from your diet, the healthier you will be. If you don't have a taste for fruit and vegetables it is probably because you have been eating mostly overcooked, overprocessed foods. Start by adding small portions a little at a time. These steps are guidelines, not hard and fast rules. Adjust them to fit you and your lifestyle.

Remember that all fried foods are hard to digest. Frying destroys a lot of the vitamins and minerals in food, not to mention what happens to oil when heated to a high temperature: some authorities say that it becomes carcinogenic. So don't make fried foods your way of life. Make your way of life the natural fresh way that God intended, and then, if you are at a restaurant or someone's home when fried food is served — or if you have been good for a month and just want a hamburger and french fries — then go ahead and enjoy it and thank God for helping you to be so good all those weeks. But *remember*, this is *not* your way of life and *not* a daily occurrence. If you're one who is not led into temptation by such things then praise God because you have a wonderful gift. Most of us are tempted and it is with great restraint, discipline, and conscious obedience to God's ways that we stay on the right track. Whatever we do only now and then in our eating habits, whether it is something good for us or something bad, won't make much difference in the long run. It's what we do every day that determines whether we will be healthy or sick.

It is important not to make your diet "meat heavy." That's the reason for the twenty-five percent limit on meat. Too much meat can be exhausting for your system to process and the result may be fatigue and weight gain. Remember, flesh foods are not as good as earth-grown foods. That doesn't mean you don't eat flesh foods, but don't overload your diet with them. I was amazed at how strong I became on a diet of fifty percent fresh fruits and vegetables. I had always believed that if I didn't have meat or chicken with every meal I would die. Now I am stronger than I've ever been, having beef only once or twice a month, and chicken, turkey, and fish once during the week.

A Word About Sprouts

Sprouts deserve a special little section because they are a unique food in that they are *living* when you eat them. In a time of disaster or food shortage, you could exist on sprouts alone. All you need are the seeds and a little sprouter and you can grow them yourself easily in a few days. I used to dislike sprouts. They made me feel like I was grazing in the field when I ate them. But then, as I began to read about them and study their worth, I found them to be a *miracle* food. They are a wonderfully pure food and you should never turn down a chance to eat them. Sprouts are digested easily and assimilated quickly; they are low in calories; extremely high in vitamins, minerals, and digestive enzymes; and you receive great physical benefits from them with very little time and effort. So, in the economy of things, sprouts seem like a very good buy. Keep them in mind.

Even You Can Love Herb Teas

I once took soft drinks and iced tea as my only drinks; I had to get used to water and then to herb teas. I at first had the feeling that with sprouts and herb teas I would close my eyes one day and turn into a rabbit. That, however, was because my jaded taste buds had been catered to in perverted ways with too many sweets. When I was put on a seven-day fast by my nutritionist, I was allowed to have herb teas on the third day. They tasted wonderful! The more I have fasted through the years, the better they taste.

Every herb tea has a soothing and healing quality to it. My favorite, and the one you probably should start with, is peppermint tea. It's a wonderful drink anytime, but especially early in the morning. When you are healthy you won't need something as strong and stimulating as coffee to get you going. A cup or two of peppermint tea will do nicely. It's also good after meals as it aids in digestion. Herbs have been used for medicine since Adam and Eve had to make it on their own. Don't be fooled in the markets by teas that are called peppermint but have an ingredients list that begins, "Tea, peppermint...." This means that it contains regular tea, with all its caffeine and acid-causing, vitamin-B depleting properties, and has an added peppermint flavoring. It must say *herb* tea on the front of the box. Other good herb teas are: Rose hip, comfrey, chamomile, and herbal laxative tea.

Foods to Avoid; Foods to Include

I have prepared two simple lists: the first gives you the most frequently consumed foods that should not be a part of a way-of-life-type eating. All foods on this foods-to-avoid list should be eliminated completely. It *can* be done because there is a satisfying replacement for each one on the list of foods to include, which follows. If you have difficulty eliminating something completely, at least try to use it sparingly.

Begin by crossing off all the foods on the foods-to-avoid list that you already avoid anyway. Next, go through the list again and check off any foods that would be no problem for you to eliminate totally from your diet right away. Now with what is left, eliminate one item each week. By eliminate, I mean throw them completely out of the house. Don't try to do it all at once, unless you're the type that can. At the same time, pick one item from the foods-to-include list and begin to include it in your diet—preferably one with the correlating number of something you have eliminated. A fast of from twenty-four to thirty-six hours just prior to each elimination or addition will help reeducate your taste buds and give you strength and new resolve to carry through.

Foods to Avoid

1. **White sugar**
2. **White-sugar products:** jams, jelly, prepared gelatin desserts, cakes, candies, cookies, pies, pudding, fruits canned in sugar, etc.
3. **White flour**
4. **White-flour products:** macaroni, noodles, spaghetti.
5. **Wheat flour:** This is usually a mixture of white and wheat. To be acceptable, it should say *whole* wheat or *stone-ground whole* wheat.
6. **Soft drinks** made with sugar and chemicals.
7. **Refined cereals**
8. **Salt and highly salted foods:** potato chips, salted nuts, pretzels, olives, etc.
9. **White rice**

10. **Hydrogenated oils and saturated fats**
11. **Peanut butter** that is highly processed and contains salt.
12. **Margarine** made from saturated fats and hydrogenated oils.
13. **Heavily processed meats:** hot dogs, salami, bologna, bacon, corned beef, etc.
14. **Canned goods** that contain white flour, sugar, or chemicals.
15. **Chocolate**
16. **Ice cream made with chemicals**
17. **Coffee, tea, and alcohol**
18. **"Instant" packaged foods**
19. **Fried foods**
20. **Canned fruits and vegetables**

Foods to Include

1. **Honey:** or at least unrefined sugar used sparingly.
2. **Foods sweetened with honey:** other good sweeteners are blackstrap molasses, fruit, fruit juice, dates.
3. **Whole-grain flour:** barley, oats, wheat, millet, rye, buckwheat, etc.
4. **Whole-grain products:** noodles, macaroni, etc., made with sesame, soya, whole wheat, artichoke, spinach.
5. **Whole-wheat flour:** or any other whole-grain flour mixture.
6. **Natural fruit juices:** If you must have soft drinks at least buy the natural ones like grapefruit soda, lemon-lime soda, sparkling apple juice, etc.
7. **Whole-grain cereals:** raw oats, four-grain cereal, whole-grain granola, etc.
8. **Avoid salt totally:** or at least salt lightly and use natural vegetable seasonings. Buy foods unsalted.
9. **Natural brown rice:** also unprocessed wild rice.
10. **Oils that are naturally pressed and unrefined:** especially sesame, corn, safflower, soya, all-blend oils.
11. **Natural peanut butter:** made without chemicals, heavy processing, and salt.
12. **Butter:** made as purely as possible.

13. **Pure meats:** look for all-meat hot dogs, bacon, etc., that are made without chemicals, sugar, preservatives, and heavy spices.
14. **Canned goods that are pure:** you should be able easily to read the labels because they list only pure natural ingredients.
15. **Carob:** many carob products are now sweetened with dates or fruit juice.
16. **Ice cream made with pure foods,** such as pure milk, eggs, and honey.
17. **Herb teas:** peppermint, rose hips, chamomile, comfrey, herbal laxative.
18. **Natural unprocessed products:** for example, if you've been buying instant potatoes, buy fresh potatoes and bake them.
19. **Baked, poached, steamed, or stewed foods:** buy a little metal vegetable steamer that fits inside your covered saucepan. It is invaluable.
20. **Fresh fruits and vegetables**

Overeating and Other Disorders

In the seven years that we have had a prayer group in our home, the most frequently voiced personal, practical prayer request from women has been for the Lord's help in controlling their eating habits and weight. I'm sure that the members who have come in and out of this group for the past seven years are typical of people everywhere. Life seems to get out of control fastest in the food department.

Millions of people are suffering with an eating disorder of some sort, the most common of which is overeating. Overeating is often the result of psychological problems and hurts. If you fall prey to this habit, try to discern the reason for it. Find out why you eat too fast, too much, between meals, when you're unhappy, when you're alone, etc. If you're hungry all the time, you are showing signs of problems other than the actual need for food. If you crave certain unhealthful foods, this is not hunger but rather a sign that something is not right inside of you. Far too many people have these problems. Food is often used to satisfy needs much greater and deeper than it was ever intended to do. People use food to help them cope with life, escape from life, deny their life, and ultimately lose their life.

Two extreme forms of obsessive eating are anorexia and bulimia. I'm not going to address these problems in this book because they would require another whole book. But I will say that if you are suffering with one of these disorders, you should put this book down and go immediately for help. Confess your situation to a parent, a friend, a pastor, a counselor, or a doctor and have them put you in touch with people who are knowledgeable about these things and can help you. Do not try to deal with it alone.

Those with less extreme obsessions should not allow themselves another moment of unbalanced eating. If you do things with food only when no one else is looking, come out of the darkness and expose those things immediately. You should examine yourself for *any* type of a secret life that you are leading. I'm not talking about letting the world know every move you make. I'm talking about having a private life of some sort where no one on earth knows or even suspects what you are doing. This can be hazardous to your health and you should proceed no further without exposing it to light. If you have a secret life, you probably have a heavy burden of guilt, too. Expose it to a pastor, a counselor, a parent, a friend, a doctor, a psychiatrist, or all of the above. This is the first step in being free. "He who conceals his sins does not prosper, but whoever confesses and renounces them finds mercy." [6]

Many of us overeat occasionally and at certain times in our lives. In times of major change, extreme stress, disappointment, busyness, or during certain illnesses we will be tempted to overeat. Remember, however, that overeating is never good for you and must not become a way of life. The worst part about it is that we usually overeat food that has no nourishment so we end up eating even more to make up for the hidden hunger or empty, incomplete feeling. Much eating is merely catering to out-of-control taste buds rather than to real hunger.

When we do overeat the body can't process the food fast enough so it ends up overtaxing the digestive organs. It

[6] Proverbs 28:13 (NIV)

makes the stomach, liver, kidneys, and bowels work harder than they are supposed to. If the food cannot be processed before it putrifies, poisons from the putrification are absorbed into the blood and the whole system is affected by dirty blood and toxic poisons. When your body has to work so hard to process all that extra food, it puts added stress on the entire system. After enough years of this the body will break down. The only way I have found to put a stop to an out-of-control appetite is through fasting (more about this in chapter 5).

Overeating uses up your energy supply. If all you feel like doing after a meal is taking a nap, it could be that you are eating too much. You need to distinguish between the feeling of being full, or stuffed, and that of being nourished and well fed. The latter is a clear-headed, energetic feeling. We don't want to live as "enemies of the cross of Christ. Their destiny is destruction, their God is their stomach, and their glory is in their shame." [7] "All a man's efforts are for his mouth, yet his appetite is never satisfied." [8]

What do your present eating habits reflect? Be realistic and honest. Are they balanced? Are they done with the glory of God in mind? Consideration of health? Appearance? Are they done out of a need? If so, what? A need for love? For comfort? To fill some emptiness inside? It's really important to your health to figure this out.

Often just having all the Seven Steps to Greater Health in order will put a stop to many eating inbalances. A person doesn't have to be overweight to be an overeater. Skinny people can overload their bodies, too, and while they may not retain weight, they do retain the effect of an overloaded system and can experience a breakdown. You can overeat good food as well as junk food. Always remember, any food that is good for you, consumed in excess, can be harmful.

Painless Weight Loss

We've gone berserk over weight loss today because thinness is fashionable. Minimal weight is "in." This attitude has people feeling like social failures if they weigh three ounces

[7] Philippians 3:18-19 (NIV)
[8] Ecclesiastes 6:7 (NIV)

more than the skinny bikini-clad models in the soft-drink advertisements. But we must get our eyes off the advertisements and onto Jesus. God loves us the same whether we are fat or thin. Satan doesn't care if you are fat or thin either, as long as you are incapacitated and can't move toward what God has for you. You can be incapacitated in a skinny body as well as a fat one. However, you will shorten your life span by staying overweight. You'll have more sickness, disease, and back and heart problems. Ask any insurance company; they'll tell you so, and it is their business to know.

Excess weight is not fun, no matter how little or great the amount is. But the biggest problem is not whether God still loves you. He does, and so do other people. Nor is the biggest problem whether you look good in your clothes. The most important thing is whether you're going to be incapacitated by fat-related diseases and die prematurely. As far as I can see, the only reasons you would want to retain excess fat is if you plan to run naked through Alaska in January (fat keeps you warm) or to rent out your body as a life raft in July (fat floats).

In general, people tend to overeat. They keep eating and eating because they are never satisfied. Their taste buds have been jaded and perverted so that they crave foods that are wrong for them. Eating devitalized food always leaves the body wanting something more because it is never supplied with all the vitamins, minerals, and digestive enzymes it needs. Between the stress we live under and the foods we eat, it isn't any wonder that there are so many diseases, chronic ailments, and problems with overweight. What we really need is *less food, better quality food,* and *simpler food* than we tend to eat now.

Most weight-loss diets are unnatural and too restricting to stay on for any length of time. No wonder they are discouraging. You can get weight off with certain diets, but keeping it off is the problem. And you can end up losing more than weight. You can lose health. That's why it's not a diet that you need, but a new way of life. You need to know God's ways and how He originally intended you to live. When you begin living on food the way God made it, you don't have to worry about going on a diet. You eat just like the rest of us but you cut down the portions of meat, grains, and dairy products and increase the portions of fruits and vegetables. You must, however, have your diet totally balanced and be eating this way for a good month before you begin to cut back. That way you will be gaining health and never losing energy or stamina as the weight drops off.

Those I have known personally who have established this naturally balanced way of eating while observing the other seven steps have lost the weight they needed to lose and gained only health. Remember, all the steps work together to balance everything out. In other words, you must be controlling stress (which causes a lot of overeating of bad food) and exercising (which is an absolute must for establishing a normal weight balance) and drinking plenty of pure water (which flushes out the system of impurities) and fasting (which controls an out-of-control appetite) and getting plenty of fresh air, sunshine, and rest (which allows the body to rebuild in a healthy, strong way). All of these things work together to balance the body; isolate one or two and the effect is lost.

Hunger does not have to be a way of life. Neither does culinary boredom. But the tastebuds do need to be humbled and re-educated to God's ways just as all the other areas of our lives do. If you are used to having colas, cookies, chocolate cakes, and potato chips every day, of course, you aren't going to be excited about beets. But if you have been fasting, a baked potato or an avocado can seem heaven-sent.

Don't let weight loss be your concern at first, let it be *good health*. Allow your body to accustom itself to this way of eating and see how it is affected. Be patient. Take it a step and a day at a time. You'll begin to feel lighter, more energetic, and clear-headed. Remember, this is the way God intended you to live in the first place—it's not a fad!

I learned the hard way that starvation diets for quick weight loss are unnatural and extremely bad for your health. With each of my two pregnancies I gained almost fifty pounds. And since I didn't give birth to forty-pound babies I had over thirty pounds to lose each time. The first pregnancy was seven years ago when I was just learning about God's ways and foolishly thought I could disobey just this once. After the baby came, I began to starve myself, skip meals, or just nibble here and there. Soon I was tired all the time and suddenly had allergies I'd never had before. I sneezed and coughed all day long and ended up with a low-grade infection in my body that took many months to heal. By the time the baby was six months old I had lost all the weight, but I looked thin, pale, and sickly, and I felt terrible. It took me a year to get back to normal.

By the time the second child was born I had learned much more of the Lord's ways than I had known five years earlier. I decided that either all the Lord has taught me was true, or it wasn't. Either what I had been teaching in my classes about losing weight would work, or it wouldn't. I don't have a problem with being disciplined, so if I am properly motivated to do something I will do it. Let me assure you that having size-sixteen hips on a size-eight body was motivation enough for me. So I began to do strictly just what I have been recommending to you. I ate a diet of fifty percent raw or properly cooked fruits and vegetables; twenty-five percent of one meal was meat, and twenty-five percent of another meal or two were whole grains of some kind. The only snacks were nuts, seeds, and berries. I ate eggs and dairy products (homemade yogurt, unprocessed cheese, kefir, and cottage cheese) only two or three times a week and only in very small portions. It was as simple as that. I also exercised five days a week for thirty to sixty minutes. When the baby was no longer nursing, I began twenty-four-hour fasts once a week. I spent time with my children in the fresh air and sun, I drank plenty of water, and I made sure I got eight hours of sleep at night. The weight began to fall off of me and I was back to my normal weight — and was healthy — by the time the baby was six months old. This took *exactly* the same amount of time as when I starved myself and ended up sick after the first pregnancy. It also proved another suspicion of mine: "baby weight" is not like other weight and you can only bring it off so fast. It's there so that you can sustain another life and it takes time for the body to let go of it. So be especially patient if you've had a baby in the last year or two.

If you eat the way God intended you to eat, excess weight will come off slowly and painlessly! But if you lost four pounds in one week and then nothing for three weeks, don't be concerned. Your body has to adjust and normalize. If you feed it right, it knows what to do to balance itself at a normal weight. If you want to lose weight a little faster (never more than two pounds a week) then all you do is cut down on the portions, always keeping the same ratio of the fifty percent fresh fruits and vegetables, etc. The body needs to make adjustments after a certain amount of weight loss before it can begin shedding weight again. It does that so that you don't deplete any area of your body. So if you come to plateaus every ten pounds or so do not be discouraged—it's a sign of health.

In her book *Free To Be Thin* Marie Chapian says, "Don't plan for failure." By hiding foods you shouldn't eat, even by bringing them into the house, you are planning for failure. And nibbles and tastes, although they seem like so little, make a difference.

Don't skip meals. If you don't like breakfast, just eat a piece or two of fruit. That is one of the best breakfasts you could have anyway. You will stay healthy and actually lose weight faster by eating three meals a day evenly spaced at five-to-six-hour intervals. When you skip meals or starve yourself to lose weight you are defeating your purpose because you put the body into a complete state of confusion and it begins to store up for famine by not allowing its reserves to go out as quickly. When you eat three meals a day the body burns calories in an even manner.

Do not think that eating God's way is restrictive. It isn't. His laws are never restrictive—they are releasing. They are there to give us a more fulfilling life. The important thing is to learn of God's ways and love them enough to make them a way of life. That's what I did and the weight came off with no pain, no sickness, no starvation, and no misery. Of course, I would have liked everything to have happened in a week, but God didn't ask us to have patience for nothing. His ways take a little more time than we would like, perhaps, but they're worth it.

Don't give up when you blow it. It doesn't matter how great the failure, just confess it to God so you don't get loaded down with guilt; keep on doing what you know is right. Above all, let your main reason for losing weight be to have a long, healthy life of service to the Lord. Fitting into your "Calvins" is not motivation enough.

If you need to lose more than forty pounds, please, please, please, find a good doctor for supervision. Don't do it out of a book. You need a good medical doctor and/or a good nutritionist, someone qualified to keep an eye on you and look for hidden danger, like high blood pressure. However, if you are more than seventy-five pounds overweight get yourself to a doctor or hospital program that specializes in weight loss. Your problems are unique, your body chemistry has changed, and you are not going to respond in the same way as someone who is just twenty to forty pounds overweight. Don't even try it alone. Seek specialized help. It *can* be done but it *must* be *done right* or else you'll end up sick, discouraged, and feeling as if you've failed when the truth will be that the problem just wasn't handled properly.

Also, please know that there is much evidence that an allergy could be at the root of an obesity problem. You could be retaining weight because of an allergic reaction to a particular food. If so, you need the help of a doctor who specializes in treating allergies. This is another good reason not to handle a serious weight problem alone. Find a good doctor.

Learning New Habits

You have two hundred sixty *trainable* taste buds. Eating habits are learned and you can teach yourself to eat any way you want. No one is born craving cola and chocolate, although you may feel certain that you are the one exception. You *learned* to love the foods you love now, and you can *learn* to love God's food just as much. I used to love cola and chocolate more than anything and I certainly had the health and appearance to prove it. But today I not only no longer crave those things, I never even think about them. They are not options. Now I feel about a baked potato, avocado, banana, or papaya the way I used to feel about a hot-fudge sundae. I changed by learning to love God's ways and by fasting and praying to break down the strongholds around my taste buds (more about this in chapter 5).

Keep It Simple

Our lives have gotten too complex and so have the foods we eat. When you can appreciate the simple, pure foods that God made, you will be much happier and healthier. You will find that you consistently feel better after meals that are simple. Fewer different types of foods, simply prepared, will be healthier for you and easier to digest. Watch for the dangers of twelve-course meals, buffets, and pot-luck dinners: we all have a tendency to think it is our God-given right to have a helping from every single dish. Choose several things that appeal to you, and make healthful, balanced choices. You'll enjoy the dinner so much more, and you'll feel better the next day.

Get rid of the idea that everything you see in the grocery store is good to eat. Much of it is not, and you have to make decisions based on knowledge and wisdom as to what you should bring into your house. Make choices that are simple. If we had to go out and milk the cow, gather the eggs, grind the grain, pick the fruit, catch the fish, or kill the chicken just to have dinner, we might be very often tempted to say, "let's pick a few potatoes, tomatoes, and ears of corn from the garden tonight and just keep it simple."

Because everything is so readily available we have either "decision anxiety" or "food overdose." Keep that in mind. To have every food you've ever dreamed of at your fingertips at every moment is not natural.

Fruits and vegetables, nuts, seeds, and whole grains are naturally grown food God made for us. The less that is done to them in the way of preparing them to be eaten, the better. When they are prepared *simply*, they will give you more strength and more health than fancy, richly prepared foods.

Daily Variety

Get yourself out of any habit of having the same food over and over every day, month in and month out. No matter what the food is this is not good for you. Whether it's butter, wheat, eggs, yogurt, carrots, milk, oranges, or meat, do not have it every day. God made things seasonal, not to be eaten every day of the year. Many foods can also become an irritant to your system if you have them every day. That doesn't mean you can't have a certain food a few days in a row if you happen to have an abundance of it, but after that give your body a break from it.

Stress-free Eating

All nutritionists agree that it doesn't make any difference how healthful the food that you eat is if you cannot digest it and assimilate it. Stress affects digestion and without good digestion you don't convert the foods you eat to something assimilable. Unless the food you eat is broken down properly, it cannot enter the rest of your body to be used as energy. The breaking down of the food begins the minute it enters your mouth. If you gulp, eat too fast, or eat under stressful conditions, you short-change this process. "Better a dry crust with peace and quiet than a house full of feasting, with strife." [9]

When you eat, set the tone of peace with your prayer of blessing upon the food. This doesn't have to be a long-winded time of intercessory prayer; a few sentences will cover it. I've always had trouble with people who sit down to eat and go on and on with such a prayer that you wonder if this is the only prayer time they've ever had. This is not the time to pray for Aunt Millie's pet snake or the dog's sore paw. This is not the time to intercede for China while the potatoes get cold. This is a brief time to focus on the Giver of all things, to thank Him for our daily bread, and to set a tone of peace and gratitude. Have a separate special prayer time for all other needs. Setting a tone of peace is important. Even if you're alone in a busy, crowded restaurant and you're not the type to pray openly in public, at least take a moment to close your eyes, breathe deeply,

[9] Proverbs 17:1 (NIV)

and say, "Thank you, Lord, for this food and your peace," and begin to eat slowly, thinking about whatever is true, honest, right, pure, lovely, admirable, excellent, or praiseworthy. It will affect your entire being. Tension is an enemy to health, especially to good eating.

All the foods on the foods-to-avoid list cause stress. They actually starve and irritate the nerves. Just by avoiding those foods and by including the ones on the foods-to-include list you will reduce the stress on your body.

Eating Out

I know what you're thinking. You fear that your social life is over and you will never be able to go out to dinner at a restaurant again. But this is not true. All you have to do is learn to make wise choices. You don't run out to Maggie's Grease Joint anymore for a cup of fried soup. You search out the places with great salad bars, and the ones that serve properly cooked vegetables and fresh fish, chicken, and meat. Avoid restaurants that cook their vegetables (which came from a can in the first place) beyond recognition. In restaurants my motto has always been, "If you can't identify it, don't eat it." More and more restaurants now serve natural brown rice and whole-grain breads. If you are in a restaurant where not everything is good, just eat what *is* good. Don't feel you have to clean your plate because of all the starving children in India. They aren't going to feel any better if you're overweight. (If you want to help the starving children in India then fast and pray for them, and send the money you would have spent on food to one of the organizations that gives them aid.) It's worth the effort to inquire about good, healthful restaurants.

When there are unavoidable times of fast foods or processed junk, you will find that you will not be harmed too much by such a meal if you have been following all of the seven steps and have made eating God's way your way of life. But don't be fooled into thinking you can get away with it all the time. "You may be sure that your sins will find you out." [10] A common error we all make when we are

[10] Numbers 32:23 (NIV)

doing well is to want to stray back to our old ways. The entire Old Testament is full of such cases.

If you are invited to someone's house, go and be thankful for whatever they serve you. If it is a buffet or pot luck you can exercise your wisdom and freedom of choice. If it's not, concentrate on what is pure healthful food and go light on what isn't. If, however, you arrive for dinner and find it's fried salami with white rice, chocolate-covered corn chips (I once heard corn chips described as a vegetable), and lollipops in a bed of powdered sugar for dessert, you could always take a few tastes of each, exclaim at its uniqueness, and tell the hostess if she just had a few carrot slices your life would be complete. What you must not do is hit your hostess over the head with your Bible and scream at her, "Don't you know about God's way of eating!" Be polite and caring about the feelings of others when it comes to eating at someone else's house. If you're really concerned about what someone might serve you, invite them to *your* house first, get together at a restaurant, do something together that doesn't require eating, or volunteer to bring the salad. At any rate, your social life is not over—that is, unless you try to convert all your friends to your way of eating!

Special Occasions

If you are eating food the way God made it as a "way of life," when it comes to special occasions you can feel free to enjoy them. For example, don't feel guilty about having a piece of your birthday cake, chocolate mousse at your anniversary dinner, pumpkin pie at Thanksgiving, Christmas cookies, or a little ham at Easter. However, do not have all those things at one meal and DO NOT GORGE! Overeating is never good—not even on special occasions. Have a calmness about food, not a desperate greediness. When you really don't have a strong desire for a certain thing, refuse it (within the bounds of politeness, of course). If your hostess goes to great lengths to prepare a dessert especially for you (and you made no mention of not eating desserts before you accepted the invitation), do not say, "I don't feel like dessert tonight, thank you." You will appear ungrateful and your hostess may be offended. Say instead,

"Yes, I would love a very small portion."

One last thing: Do not go around looking for special occasions. Celebrating Groundhog Day, Guatemalan Independence and Bob Hope's birthday all in the same week gets a little suspicious. More than one special occasion a month and you'd better start asking for mini-portions.

God's Food and Children's Stomachs

I have frequently been asked, "How do you get your children to eat food the way God made it?" Once children have already learned to love the wrong foods — and they must contend with peer pressure and attend birthday parties — re-educating them is more difficult.

I had tried my best to teach our son, Christopher, to love healthful food when he was a baby. However, many things found their way into my kitchen and my son's mouth via his junk-food-loving dad. I did my best to educate my husband and son, but they seldom listened. But since strife in a family does *far more* damage than eating junk food can do, I didn't push the matter. I would just prepare the best food I could and they would eat it, and have their soda and candy snacks at other times.

My husband began to have trouble keeping his weight down and he wasn't feeling good most of the time. When he had a physical checkup, the doctor told him he had high cholesterol. I convinced him to come with me to see a Christian nutritionist. The nutritionist put him on a strict diet of all the foods I have just told you about. He was a new person in about eight weeks. I've never seen anyone change so fast. He lost the extra weight, his eyes became bright and clear, he no longer had frequent colds, and when he went back to the doctor his cholesterol was down. He quickly became a believer in God's way of eating.

For a while, we just let Christopher continue eating in his usual way. But he was getting ear infections at least once a month. I finally took him to the same nutritionist and asked, "What should I be feeding him?" He looked at me in amazement and said in his most polite voice, "He should be eating the same things you are." What ignorance on my part — of course, he should be eating the same things we were! Did God intend all this wonderful fresh healthful food for us and refined, processed, foodless goodies for our children? Certainly not. Michael and I sat down together to talk to our three-year-old. I said, "Christopher, I have done something wrong. I have let you eat a lot of bad food and it has weakened your health. Our doctor says that if you don't want to have ear infections all the time, you need to eat like we eat—the way God made food."

Even though we had prayed about this beforehand, I wasn't prepared for the miracle that followed. He said, "Okay Mom, okay Dad," and that was it. All the changes didn't happen overnight, but the transition was much smoother than I had anticipated. When *both* parents firmly believe a certain way to be right, the child accepts it more readily. He still eats more junk than I would like, but he acquired a taste for many very healthful foods, which surprised me. He still gets a chocolate-chip cookie for dessert some nights, and he has his share of goodies at birthday parties, but he has not been sick during the past three years, and this is the biggest miracle of all. Our little girl has had a much easier time of it because she wasn't exposed to junk in the first place. She sees her big brother eating his squash and baked potato and assumes it must be the "in" thing to be doing.

I still get complaints occasionally. When I hear, "Aw, Mom! Jimmy's mother doesn't make him eat four-grain cereal in the morning. He gets doughnuts," I say, "That's because Jimmy's mom doesn't know about God's ways and that they are good." When I hear, "Why do you always make me eat my vegetables?" I say, "I do that because I love you so much and I care what happens to you." He may still prefer fast-food french fries to my vegetables but he loves the fact that I said that. It makes him feel secure to know that we are looking out for his interests. Besides, he gets his fast-food hamburgers now and then, gets a gooey chocolate junk cake for his birthday, and has a big root-beer float when we go to Disneyland. But that's not his way-of-life-type eating. He knows that, and he knows why, and this makes those special treats all the more special. I wish I had known as much when I was seven.

The main rule is that if you don't want children to eat certain foods, don't bring those foods into the house. Be reasonable, understanding, and patient. Just prepare God's fresh food the best way you know how and don't allow mealtime to be a stressful time. That does more damage than junk food.

Vitamins

Doctors say that if you eat·properly you don't need food supplements or vitamins. I agree, but the problem is eating properly. It's not easy to get fresh natural food undepleted and have a totally balanced diet all the time. Food is picked prematurely and artificially ripened. That's not the way God intended it, and something is lost. Besides improper cooking and processing, there are many reasons why you might not be getting all the nutrients you require.

If you do take vitamins, be sure they too are natural and pure. Remember, you get what you pay for, and vitamins are no exception. If you buy the cheapest brand, believe me, they're not worth much. I'm not saying you have to spend a fortune, but do check the labels. Make sure they say that the vitamins are natural and without added chemicals. Buy reliable brands that have been around for a while or that are recommended by people you know. One *good* vitamin is worth fifty cheapies.

Don't ever try to live on supplements by themselves. In other words, don't eat all the junk you want and then make up for the nutrients you are missing by taking vitamins. That does not work. Vitamins are not food the way God made it no matter how natural they are. Man makes alfalfa tablets, for example, and God made alfalfa sprouts. You will always be better off eating sprouts than you will be taking pills. It's just wisdom that if you eat things as close to the way God made them as possible, you save yourself a lot of problems. You can take too many pills, but I have never seen anyone take an overdose of sprouts. Vitamins are food supplements, not substitutes. If you travel a lot and are subject to "who-knows-what-from-God-only-knows-where" food, vitamins might be a good idea. But remember, vitamins will never replace food or make up for poor eating habits.

Labels

You have to be aware of what you are putting into your body. Read all labels and be suspicious if you cannot understand them. The word "natural" on a product may mean that the food has undergone only limited processing and that no chemicals, preservatives, or colorings have been added. The word natural doesn't guarantee healthful food, however. "Organic" means that the food was grown without chemicals, pesticides, and fertilizers. When reading labels my motto has always been, "If you can't understand the label, don't eat it."

What Affects Diet and Appetite

You don't have the same appetite or nutritional requirements when the weather is warm as you do when it's cold. In the winter you may need hot, hearty soups, meats, and breads, and in the summer require only fresh fruit and vegetables. If you live in a cold climate you will need more substantial food. If you live in a warm climate, you'll want to eat lightly and flesh foods may seem too heavy.

The amount of food we eat should be determined by how much physical energy we expend. For example, if you are a secretary and sit all day using only your head and your hands, you will need to be especially careful not to overeat and what you do eat must be of high nutritional quality. On the other hand, if you are working outdoors in hard physical labor, you will need to eat more and you may eat liberally, providing that the food you eat is natural and whole.

You may have preferences for certain cuisines, such as Italian, Oriental, French, or regional American. But know that in each of these, there are certain things that God made common to all. Fruits, vegetables, berries, nuts, seeds, whole grains, fish, poultry, red meats, eggs, honey, and milk products.

Helpful Hints

1. When choosing food always ask yourself, "Is this man-made or God-made?" and "How pure can I get it?

2. The fewer items in a meal, the less you are tempted to overeat and the easier it is to digest.
3. The more natural the food, the more healthful it is, and the harder it is for you to overeat.
4. The less active your life or work, the less you need to eat.
5. Space your eating to put five or six hours between each meal. A good schedule would be breakfast at seven, lunch at noon or one, and dinner at six or seven. A bad schedule is breakfast at eleven, lunch at half-past one, and dinner at ten.
6. Eliminate one or two foods from the foods-to-avoid list every week and add from the foods-to-include list.
7. Don't eat overcooked or processed foods.
8. Eat foods ripe and in season.
9. Drink water, herb teas, and freshly squeezed juices.
10. Don't eat fried food.
11. Eat simply and plainly.
12. Never overeat.
13. Chew well.
14. Read labels.
15. Fifty percent of every meal should consist of raw or properly cooked fruits and vegetables.

God's Way—A Way of Life

The more you know about God's food and His intended way for us to grow it, prepare it, and eat it, the easier it will be for you to make this your way of life—and that is what it must become. You can't just have a cup of herb tea and an alfalfa sprout and expect that to do it for you. God's way of eating is a way of life and when you love God's ways and know that they are good, it's easy to walk in them. If you keep your refrigerator and pantry full of foods the way God made them, then when you want a meal or just a snack, you'll eat well. You may have to go to the grocery store twice a week instead of once, but that's a small price to pay. Think what that extra hour or two a week means when you stack it up against a two-month hospitalization for some disease that could have been prevented by eating God's way.

Be secure in what you know of the way God made food. Don't jump on any food-fad bandwagon (there will always be one). If you read in some article that "a candy bar a day keeps the doctor away" (God didn't make candy bars), or "green peppers for breakfast each morning will help your sex life" (unbalanced), or "instant sprouts — just add water and stir" (too far removed from the way God made sprouts), or "research has found that you need every kind of food available every day in order to stay alive" (lacks simplicity), "being fat protects you from the effects of smog" (dumb), you should be able confidently to say, "Lord, I thank you that you have shown me your ways for eating. I know your ways are good and I can trust them."

If you determine to live life free of the effects of stress by always being in touch and in tune with your Creator, eating food the way God made it, observing regular times of fasting and prayer, flushing your body free of impurities by drinking plenty of pure water, getting daily exercise, fresh air, sunshine, and deep peaceful rest at night, your body will rebuild itself in such a way that you will be truly healthy, youthful, attractive, and alive.

Words of Truth

*"Don't you know that you are God's temple and
that God's Spirit lives in you? If anyone
destroys God's temple, God will destroy him."*
I Corinthians 3:16-17 (NIV)

*"For such people are not serving our Lord Christ,
but their own appetite."*
Romans 16:18 (NIV)

*"Turn my eyes away from worthless things;
renew my life according to Your word."*
Psalm 119:37 (NIV)

*"Everything is permissible—
but not everything is beneficial."*
I Corinthians 10:23 (NIV)

*"But put on the Lord Jesus Christ, and make no
provision for the flesh, to fulfill its lust."*
Romans 13:14 (NKJ)

*"Let us purify ourselves from everything that
contaminates body and spirit, perfecting
holiness out of reverence for God."*
II Corinthians 7:1 (NIV)

*"So whether you eat or drink, or whatever you do,
do it all for the glory of God."*
I Corinthians 10:31 (NIV)

CHAPTER 3

Step Three: Proper Exercise

Do you make use of an automatic washing machine instead of going down to the river to wash your clothes on the stones? Do you fill your bathtub from a faucet instead of going out to the well to draw water? Do you drive to work instead of riding a horse or walking? Do you go to a grocery store for milk, bread, and vegetables instead of milking your cow, grinding your grain, and tending your garden? If you answered yes to any of these questions, you have simply been taking advantage of modern conveniences. And there is nothing in the world wrong with using modern conveniences *if* you are replacing the physical labor you've lost with some form of exercise.

We have over six hundred muscles in our body, and the rule about muscles is you either *use* them or *lose* them. In other words, if they never get any exercise, you may go to use them one day and they won't be there for you. You will have done serious damage to yourself, damage that could have been avoided. You are either building your body or tearing it down by what you do every day. And because we are such sitters—we sit to travel, to work, and to be entertained—it is all the more important that we do something to exercise those muscles we seldom use.

Nutrition specialists say that three things shorten people's lives: too much stress, poor eating habits, and lack of exercise. Medical doctors agree that the three most important contributions to health are rest, nutrition, and exercise. In fact, all health professionals rank exercise as one of our most indispensable requirements.

When it comes to exercise there are three types of people: people who do nothing; people who are obsessed with exercise and have made it their life; and people who lead active lives, not lives devoted to activity. God never intended us to be the first two types; but rather, that we all should be balanced, like the third type. If you belong to the third type, rejoice! If you belong to the second type and live a life devoted to exercise, you need to get more of Jesus into your life and you'll balance out fine. If you belong to the first type, you must consider making some very important changes, changes that begin with your attitude.

An Attitude of Activity

In your mind, do you think of yourself as living life in a reclining chair? Are the high points of your days eating and sleeping? Do you need a nap after every snack? If you miss an hour of sleep at night is the rest of your day spent planning how you can get it back? Do you become out of breath just getting up from your chair to turn off the television? Was the last time you took a walk on your wedding day when you came down the aisle? Are you living life as an observer and *never* as a doer? Do you always take the easy way out as opposed to the way that is good for you? Do you wake up in the morning angry because you must get up, instead of being thankful that you woke up at all? Do you never lead because it is so much easier to follow? Is the reason you seldom suggest going anywhere because you're afraid someone will say yes? Do you find being depressed more enjoyable than an aerobics class? Do you not invite people into your home because the effort seems too great? Does it seem like your life is wasting away and you never get anything done, or do you think, because of your unique ministry and abundance of spiritual gifts and talents, that you are exempt from this one step?

If you answered yes to any of these questions, you need to get your attitude in shape and then, most certainly, your body, too. You need to begin to see yourself as an important part of life, its movement, and its flow. If you've been thinking of yourself as a kind of nameless blob that sits around waiting for someone else to change the channel of circumstances on the television of your life, you have been listening to the wrong voice. You've been listening to the voice of your enemy (the father of lies) instead of the voice of God (the author of life). You need to know that God doesn't make nameless blobs; He makes active, vital people who *live* life. The reason for your inactivity could be illness, extreme fatigue, overweight, or habit. Whatever it is, it can all be changed. And the change must begin with your attitude. You must know that you were not made to do nothing.

Not Made To Do Nothing

God did not intend for us to sit all day under artificial light, breathing stale air, feeding on coffee and doughnuts. He did not intend for us to ride everywhere and never walk. We were not made to exercise our brains only; our bodies were meant to be used, too. When we don't use our abilities, we begin to lose them.

By not getting any exercise at all, you are a candidate for back problems, poor posture, overweight, overeating, bone disease, insomnia, chronic fatigue, varicose veins, high cholesterol, frequent headaches, hypertension, heart problems, constipation, digestive problems, stiff joints, aches and pains, poor circulation, depression, and arthritis. All of these ailments can almost always be minimized by regular exercise.

Physical inactivity also results in premature aging. In his book *Building Health and Youthfulness*, Paul Bragg says, "as little as thirty minutes of intelligent exercise each day can retard the aging process ten years." We can't stop aging but we can stop *premature* aging by exercising, especially in conjunction with the other Seven Steps to Greater Health. Consistent physical exercise will help you to strengthen and tone your muscles, cleanse your body of impurities, and retard the aging process.

Studies are now showing that five out of every ten deaths are premature, and that a high percentage of people as early as their forties or fifties are exhibiting signs of old age. There is a definite trend toward premature aging and premature death, and a lack of exercise is one of the major causes.

It's obvious that regular exercise is a part of the way we are supposed to live. We don't have to look forward to loss of our mental faculties, to sickness, frailty, pain, immobility, or uselessness. We were not created to live that way. In fact, if you search deep inside to find out who you specifically were created to be and what you were created to do, you are certain to discover that you were not created to do nothing. When you make that discovery and are convinced of its truth, it will affect your whole life.

Exercise Impurities Away

All exercise helps the body to do three extremely important things: eliminate poisons, increase circulation, and strengthen muscles. Without exercise, impurities cannot be eliminated as they should, the blood does not circulate well, internal organs become inactive, and unused muscles atrophy. These are the main reasons you should desire to get adequate physical exercise.

When you are engaged in any form of exercise, you breathe deeply and inhale more oxygen. This oxygen enters the bloodstream through tiny blood vessels in the lungs. The heart pumps more blood, which carries this oxygen to the rest of the body. Toxins and waste products in the form of carbon dioxide are removed from the bloodstream at that time and expelled back through the lungs during exhalation. The more oxygen in your body, the purer the bloodstream. Remember, "life is in the blood" and good health is in a clean bloodstream. When the blood is clean, disease cannot breed there. One of the main reasons to exercise is that poisons and toxic wastes are flushed from the system by that process. The older you get, the more you need to be careful not to be inactive. When your body processes slow down, a buildup of toxic waste can make you a candidate for disease.

Exercising is also the key to good circulation. When the blood does not circulate well, internal organs do not function as well as they should. For example, if the kidneys are not functioning as they should, the breakdown and removal of uric acid is hindered and this means that there will be certain toxins that are not completely eliminated from the system.

Because circulation is greatly increased through exercise, exercise causes more oxygenated blood to travel to the brain. Since the brain affects every organ, it stands to reason that feeding it properly will be of benefit to the entire body. Endorphins, which are substances in the brain that have been found to reduce pain and produce euphoric feelings, are directly affected by exercise. Endorphin levels rise after exercise and this could be the reason that menstrual cramps and other painful problems are lessened or eliminated altogether when regular exercise becomes a part of one's life.

Besides eliminating toxic waste and increasing circulation, exercise strengthens the heart muscle. The heart can't function without oxygen. When the heart muscle is weak, it cannot pump blood as it should. But when you exercise, you strengthen the heart muscle and it can pump more blood. Did you know that your heart has to beat harder and faster when you are out of shape than it does when you are physically in good condition? In other words, a healthy heart is able to pump more blood with fewer beats than an unhealthy heart.

The main reason to exercise is for your health. Without good health you cannot do *all* the Lord has for you to do and you cannot be *all* the Lord wants you to be. I didn't say you couldn't do anything. That is not true. If you have poor health, you can still love others, pray, worship, minister, create, write, speak, and work, but you can't do them as fully as you could if you were well. Wouldn't you rather be well? Wouldn't you rather have clean blood, and a healthy, strong body that doesn't let you down when you need it. Wouldn't you rather be out helping others than home in bed nursing your cold, your allergy, your bad back, or in general catering to your lazy, sluggish, fatigued body? Of course you would! Think of exercise as an irreplaceable method for ridding your body of the impurities and weaknesses that could make you an invalid. You owe it to God and those who love you to see to it that you are healthy.

Strength of the Well-Toned Body

Have you ever hesitated to give someone your shoulder to cry on because you're afraid they might dislocate it? Have you resisted washing the feet of others because last time you did a deep knee bend you weren't able to get up for three weeks? Was there ever a time when you decided against giving someone the shirt off your back because you feared you might have a muscle spasm taking it off? There is a lot to be said for having a body with strength and flexibility. If the ligaments that link one bone to another are kept flexible, you can move freely and your body won't fail you when you need it most. You lose elasticity in the muscles, joints, and connective tissue when you don't use them. If your muscles are strong, they will hold your bones and internal organs in their proper place. If your muscles are weak, they don't hold anything in place and you end up with bad posture, which gives way to stooped shoulders, hunched back, hanging head, curvature of the spine, protruding stomach, swayback, and weak hips. This leads the way to frequent sprains, strains, pains, pulls, and dislocations.

Many of these problems begin with bad posture. To have good posture you must have a clean system that is well-nourished and properly exercised. Often people are just too chronically fatigued to stand or sit up straight, so their bodies need to be cleansed, fed well, and exercised to give them strength. Good posture also encourages your internal organs to stay in their proper place and to work more efficiently.

The strength of the body depends upon the heart, and what affects the heart—spiritually, emotionally, and physically—affects all. When your heart doesn't work properly, it does not pump as much blood as it should and the entire body is affected. The heart can be trained and strengthened, like any other muscle. In fact, one of the main reasons for exercising is to strengthen the heart.

Millions of people suffer from back problems. While a specific thing, like a turn, reach, or twist, may bring on the back problem, this is usually only the straw breaking the camel's back. You can be sure that the problem has been building for a long time. Stress, overweight, and a lack of exercise sets you up for back injury. Seventy-five percent of people with chronic back problems do not exercise and have not exercised for years. Most of them also carry extra weight. If you're not exercising and you're carrying excess weight, your stomach muscles will be weak and your posture will suffer. This puts a strain on your back and eventually it will not be able to hold up under all the mistreatment. Extra weight and no exercise is an invitation to bad back problems.

When your body is exercised, toned, strengthened, flexible, and strong, your possibilities for serving others increase. With strong, well-toned shoulder and arm muscles, you can carry grandma's suitcase up to her room when she comes to visit, instead of *her* carrying *you* in from the car because you threw your back out trying to open her door. With well-developed leg, calf, thigh, and buttock muscles you can walk that extra mile with your neighbor without collapsing and having to tell him to go on by himself. The possibilities for ministry are endless when you have a body that won't fail you.

Organized Exercise

"For bodily exercise profits little but godliness is profitable for all things having the promise of the life that now is and of that which is to come." [1]

This Scripture is the one that prompted me to make my first exercise tape and to begin teaching exercise classes. Jesus taught that spiritual food has greater value than physical food, but He never said that we should stop eating. By the same token, in comparison with spiritual exercise, bodily exercise profits little, but that doesn't mean you shouldn't get any. It just means that it should be placed in proper perspective in our lives. To ignore good nutrition and proper exercise as a way of life is foolish. Equally foolish is to put such importance upon these things that you become a slave to them. That's bondage. There must be a balance.

Everyone needs to exercise, regardless of age, size, or

[1] I Timothy 4:8 (NKJ)

shape. What will differ among individuals will be the type of exercise that appeals to them and suits their lifestyle. There is much to be said for *regular* vigorous exercise if you want to see and feel results. Regular exercise makes you healthy, youthful, attractive, and alive, and it's a great fixer for a life that feels out of control. Regular exercise strengthens your muscles, builds a stronger heart, increases your endurance.

Research has found that there are definitely fewer incidents of heart disease and strokes among people who are regular, vigorous exercisers. We now know that not only will you live longer if you exercise regularly, you will also have a better quality of life.

Suppose you agree that you want to have all of these things we have talked about—a stronger heart, more flexibility, firmer muscles, greater endurance, superior health, etc.—and suppose you are convinced that regular exercise is the way to achieve them. Now the thing to do is to get organized. You have to have a plan.

The practical approach to physical exercise is to schedule it. Just as in chapter 1 when we wrote into our datebook time for prayer and Bible reading (the spiritual exercises), you need to set aside a specific period of time each day for physical exercise. You must keep that time just as you would any other important date. Stay with it no matter what. Trying to squeeze it in at various times during the day creates an inconsistency and tends to work against discipline. If you don't *make* room for a specific thing in your schedule, you won't *have* room for it. Sit down and decide the five *W*'s: who, what, where, when, and why.

Who: Decide whether you want to exercise alone or would be better off committing yourself to something with a friend. Either way is great.

What: Decide exactly what you are going to do. It could be an aerobics class, dance class, bicycle riding, swimming, jogging, rebounding, fast walking, or whatever other vigorous, healthful exercise appeals to you. You should enjoy what you are doing or at least try to cultivate a liking for it. To do that, you need to give it a little time. If you get bored with the same exercise record, have three or four different ones. If you get tired of walking or running along a certain path, try a new area. If you become bored by your regular exercise class, try a slow-stretch class, a dance class, or an aerobics class. Whatever you decide to do, if you are not taking a class, buy a book and find out how to do it correctly so you won't hurt yourself. Even something as simple as wearing improper shoes while jogging can cause great problems in a very short time. Personally, I most enjoy working out in a class situation because it's good to have an instructor, it's inspiring to see others working, it's beneficial to observe your posture and movements in front of a mirror, and I find I work harder if someone is yelling at me. My husband, on the other hand, finds exercise more enjoyable in a game such as tennis. It doesn't matter what it is as long as you enjoy it and you do it consistently.

When choosing your form of physical exercise, it's important to think in terms of developing the whole body as opposed to just one specific area. In other words, if you have a flabby stomach, don't think in terms of doing *only* stomach exercises. That is unbalanced. Always exercise the whole body as much as you are able. If you have medical problems like a bad back, problem knees, weak ankles, a heart condition, high blood pressure, more than forty pounds overweight, or whatever, check with your doctor as to what exercises you can or should be doing. If you are out of shape and have not exercised for years, get a clearance from your doctor for your new program. Exercise will help just about any condition, provided you are doing the right kind of exercises for you.

When: Decide how many times a week you are going to exercise and at what time each day. Don't wait to see whether you feel like it in the morning. That will never work because chances are good you won't feel like it. "Feeling like it" is not a good indication of whether you *should* exercise. Never argue with yourself over this matter — decide beforehand when you are going to exercise and do it. *Schedule your exercise time.* Which times you choose are not important as long as they are *consistent* and *regular.* Write down in your datebook the exact days and times that you can do it. You need to schedule something at least three times a week (every other day) for at least twenty to thirty minutes each time (preferably an hour). Doing a strenuous sport or exercise class only once a week is too defeating. You will never build yourself up. It needs to be at least three times a week. That way you're not always breaking yourself in. As for the time of day, this is an individual preference also. Some people are better in the afternoon or early evening while others, like me, are definitely early-morning types. In fact, if I don't exercise before noon it isn't going to happen. My husband and I have worked out a routine whereby three mornings a week I drop off my son at school, take an exercise class, and return home in time for my husband to leave for work. On the other days, he takes him to school and then plays tennis with a friend. We find that when we don't do that we are grumpy, sluggish, and lazy. We're convinced it's worth the effort to get up early and exercise even if we've been up late the night before. On days I don't go to class, I use my own "Exercise for Life" tape in the morning before breakfast. If you are going to exercise first thing in the morning, you need to spend a little more time warming up and waking your sleepy body. Don't find out the hard way (like I did), by leaping out of bed right into vigorous exercise and pulling a muscle. The best way is to get up, drink two glasses of water (step four), spend time in reading and prayer with the Lord (step one), and by then your muscles will be more awake and ready to go. If you work, perhaps you could go to a gym on your lunch hour. See how refreshed and energetic you feel for the remainder of the day. Many people like to exercise in the evening because it relieves all tension and they say it helps them sleep better at night. For those of you with small children or other reasons to stay at home, trampolines, jump ropes, or exercise albums come in very handy. But you can't fall into the trap of thinking you don't need to schedule it. You do, more than anyone, because if your time isn't somewhat structured, certain very important things that you want to accomplish will never happen.

Where: You need to decide if you are going to exercise in your home or somewhere else. If it's going to be somewhere else, decide specifically where. Join a gym, check out a place to run, book a tennis court, or whatever you need to do to get access to the facilities you need.

Why: If you need to be reminded why you are exercising, reread the "forty good reasons to get up and do it" near the end of this chapter. Unless you've lost all touch with reality, somewhere in the list you should get inspired.

Always start slowly, build up gradually, and don't ever push beyond what you are able to do. In fact, find a good balance between pushing yourself too hard and not pushing yourself enough to make a difference. Whenever you stop exercising for more than a week or two, always ease back into it slowly. If you are really out of shape when you begin exercising, you may experience shortness of breath, weakness, dizziness, nausea, lack of muscle control, lightheadedness or tightness in the chest. If these occur, lighten up on what you are doing. You may be moving too fast in your program or pushing too hard. Learn to distinguish between the good pain that comes with healthy use of a muscle and the bad pain that is a sign of injury. Always stop what you are doing if something *seems* to be wrong, because you can pull a muscle without feeling pain immediately. You'll just sense that something is not right. (These things won't tend to happen if you always warm up thoroughly.)

The abdominal muscles are the most difficult to firm and will be the last ones to get into shape on an out-of-shape person just beginning an exercise program. So do not look at your tummy every day in the mirror and decide too soon that the exercises aren't working. Allow time for the abdominal muscles to become strong. This is especially true if you've had a baby. If you have had more than one child, please be patient with your tummy. It's been through a lot and it takes awhile. It will seem for a long time that nothing is happening, but don't give up because eventually those abdominal muscles will be strong.

Music always makes exercising easier. I carry my tape

recorder and exercise tape with me when we travel, and my husband and I use at least part of it every morning. This helps us to hold up better throughout the trip.

If you are stiff and sore after exercising, don't stop. Keep your schedule going and you'll work through the soreness. Start-and-stop exercising is not good because that way you never get past the sore stage.

Make sure that you stop eating one hour before you exercise. Your blood goes to the stomach to digest food, and then it must be drawn away to carry oxygen to the muscles when you exercise. One of the two will suffer if you eat and exercise too closely together.

You can expect results on a regular exercise program. But for many of you, it's best if you're not running to a scale, a mirror, or a chart to see if you're measuring up on a daily basis. For those who love a challenge, this is no problem, but it can be very destructive for some people. Learn to keep your mind and heart focused on Jesus and obediently living His way. Pretty soon you'll notice that you are feeling better and stronger, and your clothes are fitting more attractively. Just keep doing what you know is right without checking up on yourself too frequently. We're looking for a change in attitude and lifestyle. When organized exercise is a way of life, the results are sure to be there. They just don't come overnight. And don't look for any shortcuts because there aren't any that don't carry a price.

Aerobics

Aerobics has become widely popular — and for good reason. The word aerobic literally means "able to live, grow, or be active only where oxygen is present." An aerobic exercise is any very rigorous and nonstop exercise that conditions the heart and lungs by increasing oxygen intake. Aerobic exercises work the heart muscle, making it stronger and causing it to pump more oxygenated blood throughout the system. It also causes your metabolism to speed up and burn calories — a condition that will last from twenty-four to forty-eight hours after you stop exercising, so if you have an aerobics class on Monday, Wednesday, and Friday for example, you will be burning calories during almost all of the week. The leaner you become the more this will apply, because lean tissue has more oxygen in it than fat tissue does. Besides the standard aerobics class, other aerobic-type activities are swimming, bicycling, jump rope, jogging, walking at a fast pace, or rebounding (jumping on a mini-trampoline).

In one hour of aerobics three times a week, you can increase your endurance greatly; develop strong muscles; relieve pain, stress, tension, and depression; prevent constipation; improve your sleep; clear your mind; and elevate the beta-endorphic levels in the blood. Who couldn't use that kind of help? Aerobics are a very quick, concentrated way to exercise your entire body thoroughly.

Keep Breathing

One of the most important aspects of exercising is the fact that it helps you to breathe properly and causes you to breathe deeply. Because exercise improves your posture this encourages good breathing habits even when not exercising. That's why it is essential that you remember to keep breathing while engaging in any form of exercise. Don't ever hold your breath. When you do that, you don't take in enough oxygen and you don't expel enough impurities. Remember, we are breathing to keep our blood clean. When you breathe you are cleaning your system. You take in through the lungs oxygen that goes into the blood and you exhale carbon dioxide. You breathe in life, you exhale disease and death.

Muscles do not function well without air and they need even *more* oxygen when they are worked hard. If you work yourself too hard, you will require more oxygen than your heart can manage to give you. Overweight people breathe heavily because they cannot get enough oxygen to all the extra fat cells with only normal-size lungs. Your lung size doesn't increase with your body size. That's why there is such an exhausting strain on the heart when it has to pump oxygenated blood to one hundred extra pounds.

If you are exercising and get a sharp pain, or "stitch," in your side, this could be because you are holding your breath or breathing shallowly. Doctors say it is a cramp in the diaphragm muscle that happens as a result of waste buildup due to inadequate oxygenation, that is, when the blood does not pick up oxygen and drop off carbon dioxide fast enough. This can also happen when you're out of shape, if you're exercising in hot and humid weather or in a room where one hundred other people are exercising vigorously and there is inadequate ventilation. In each of these instances you are not getting enough oxygen. When you do get a side pain, the best thing to do is stop exercising and breathe slowly and deeply until it stops.

More to Life than Aerobics Class

Everyone is an individual and what appeals to some may not necessarily seem good to all. If you know for sure that you are not an organized exerciser and that you would never enroll in an aerobics class, take heart. You are not necessarily lazy, you are not odd, you are not even "out of it." You are just different. As personality expert Florence Littauer says in her book *Personality Plus*, "just because [someone] is different doesn't make [them] wrong." If you know that your image of yourself does not include bouncing around in a class with leg warmers and leotards then lift your head high, for you are in good company. I can think of quite a long list of very respectable, intelligent, reasonable people who fit into this category.

There is no record in Scripture that Jesus ever took an aerobics class. There is also no record of Him being sick, and if you will notice carefully, He did every one of the seven steps. He certainly had a right relationship with God. He ate food the way God made it. He drank plenty of pure water. He fasted and prayed. We know He spent time in fresh air and sunshine as the Gospels tell how He was often outside ministering to people. And He rested so deeply that even a storm did not wake Him. As for exercise, Jesus was a walker. He walked everywhere – uphill, downhill, to the sea, to the wilderness, and back.

Walker arise! Don't be embarrassed in this day of aerobic classes to say that you are indeed a walker. I don't care if the whole world bows down and worships the god of leotards, tights, and leg warmers, you can hold your head up high without shame. You are in good company. Walking at a vigorous pace increases your pulse rate, which means you are exercising your heart and your circulation will benefit greatly from it. It also causes you to breathe deeply. When you are walking, be sure to hold your head high, not only because you are a respectable exerciser, but because it aligns your posture. Keep your chest up, breathe deeply, and take big steps.

Some people enjoy running, which is done for speed. Some people love jogging, which doesn't take into account how long it takes to go a certain distance, but rather the distance traveled. Swimming is said to be one of the best all around exercises because it works every main muscle group in your body and forces you to breathe deeply, slowly, and with control.

Some of you might enjoy a mini-trampoline (or re-bounder, as it is now called). It's fun, it doesn't take up much space, and everyone in the family can enjoy it. It's actually a good way to begin exercising because you get a lot of benefit with just a little effort. It is about thirty-six inches in diameter and low to the ground. You can jog, bounce, or dance on it. I've heard of people who were so infirm that they couldn't stand and jump on a rebounder, but were told just to sit on it and bounce up and down. This accomplished so much in the way of exercise and stimulation to the bones, organs, and muscles that they began to improve rapidly and steadily.

Bicycling is another good form of exercise, and so are baseball, hiking, handball, and horseback riding. Never think that just because you are sitting on a horse and he appears to be doing most of the work that you're not getting a workout. You're using practically every muscle in your body to keep good balance and control. Not only that, the stimulation to the bones, organs, and muscles works just the same as on the rebounder, but much more so.

Everyone enjoys certain activities more than others. Don't feel bad if you hate to jog but love to swim, or if you've never liked swimming but enjoy bicycling, as long as you are happy doing what you are doing. You don't have to take an aerobics class, but you do have to do something.

Leading an Active Life

When you establish an attitude of activity, and go on to add a regular program of exercise at least three times a week, you begin to feel more and more like leading an active life. In an active life, it is natural to enjoy some form of physical activity daily. The best way to change your lifestyle is to go step by step. In this case, I mean that literally. Begin by walking wherever you can. Look forward to it. Rejoice in it. Be excited about it. Park a few blocks away from the restaurant and walk there. Climb up and down the stairs rather than using an elevator (unless, of course, you live on the top floor of the World Trade Center and are bringing in your groceries). When you need to have a private talk with a friend, go for a walk to do it. If you have an important problem to solve, go outside for a stroll. In just a short ten minutes you can get a sufficient supply of oxygen to the brain, allowing you to think clearly enough to solve just about any problem. Look for opportunities to travel on foot instead of driving. This takes the pressure off having to find a parking place right out in front of the post office or trying to squeeze your Lincoln Continental into a Honda-size parking space. (Walk only where you are sure it is safe, however. Accidents and muggings are not compatible with stress-free living.)

Try walking as a family affair. Sometimes after dinner my husband will organize the whole family for a walk up and down the hills near our house. He says getting everybody's shoes and jackets on for the trek is twice as much exercise as the actual walk itself. I must admit that the preparation can sometimes take longer than the walk when you have little ones, but it is worth it. When we get back we feel great and everybody sleeps well at night.

I used to be a totally inactive person. What changed me were the Seven Steps to Greater Health. The healthier and stronger I became, the more I felt like doing things. The more things I did, the more I wanted to do. The more active I became, the less inactivity appealed to me. It was miraculous. If it can happen to me, it can definitely happen to you, too!

One new way of thinking is to plan social events around some kind of physical activity. Set a date to jog three mornings a week with your husband, tell your son you'll play ball with him on Saturday, go for a walk after dinner with a neighbor, bicycle around the block with your daughter, invite your friends to go swimming on the weekend, take a friend hiking in the mountains. Knowing that someone else is depending on you motivates you on days when you might want just to sit in the television chair and eat chocolates. It's a new way of thinking.

Tension is greatly relieved by living an active life. It doesn't have the chance to build up like it does when you are inactive. Even a few stretches and deep-breathing exercises throughout the day make a difference. Remember, *everything you do counts*. You don't want to be sluggish, lazy, and barely moving. God did not create you to be that way and you don't have to settle for it.

Outdoor activity is the best, but if you can't get out of the house just put on some joyful, uplifting music and jog, jump, skip, dance, sway, or stretch to it. Try this in the place of a midmorning snack sometime. When your children are boisterous, loud, and generally driving you crazy, just put that type of music on the stereo and invite them to move with you. It will soothe their little spirits and put focus into their activity instead of frenzy. Most likely, it will end up changing the whole mood and outlook of everyone involved.

If you're a television watcher, substitute some action on television for some action in your life. Replace one program a day with some form of vigorous physical activity.

When you are on vacation, try to find activities that you don't get to do at home—horseback riding, jogging on the beach, snorkeling, riding the waves, hiking in the mountains, or just plain sightseeing walks. When traveling, plan for activity. Even if it's a business trip, be ready for unexpected exercise possibilities. Always take along swimwear, a jogging suit, or some kind of loose-fitting, all-purpose sport outfit, and a pair of tennis shoes. You never know when you might have the opportunity to use them.

Do you have grandchildren or nephews and nieces that you need to get to know better. Do something active with them. They will enjoy it and probably end up thinking, "Boy, Grandma Nancy is sure fun," or "I can't wait to see Aunt Suzy again soon." Physical activity makes you more energetic, youthful, fun, and attractive to other people — especially to teenagers and children.

There will be many times when you won't feel like getting up to do something, but you'll always be glad you did. The more good things you do for your physical body the fewer bad things you will be tempted to do. If you are just too tired to do *anything* and you're having trouble sleeping, possibly it's because you are in need of a cleansing fast. Carefully check your diet, stress level, and water, fresh air, and sunshine supply. In other words, go over all of the seven steps and see where you could be doing better in each area.

Begin immediately to change your lifestyle slowly. Begin to think active. Your muscles were made to be used. You were not created to do nothing. Activity is normal — inactivity is not. Don't wait to hear bad news from the doctor to do something. Every day you should be active or have planned some kind of physical activity. By learning to be active you create more energy and with more energy you become more active. But you have to start somewhere. You have to take the first step. Begin to let activity be a way of life.

You're Not a Lost Cause

I know that some of you are thinking, "There's no way my body can bounce up and down on a tennis court, baseball diamond, olympic diving board, or aerobics classroom floor. I'm overweight and it's an effort for me just to get out of bed in the morning. I'm a lost cause when it comes to exercise." Most of the people who feel like lost causes suffer from overweight and have not yet found the key to making their bodies balanced and whole again. I have counseled and prayed with many a person in agony over this problem and I deeply sympathize with the intense frustration and hopelessness that often accompanies it. But let me assure you that I have seen wonderful, almost miraculous results in many extremely overweight people who were able to discover God's plan for their lives and see how He intended them to live. Most of them did seek the help of a doctor or specialist in the field of health or weight loss, but in every case that had lasting results, *none* of the laws of God were violated. In other words they were not given fad diets, strange concoctions, or unusual methods. In every case I can think of where a person went on a diet totally different from the way of life I am speaking about in this book, the weight loss was temporary and they eventually went back to the way they were. Some of them ended up in a worse condition because they lost more than weight, they also lost their health. Remember: THERE ARE NO SHORTCUTS TO HEALTHY WEIGHT LOSS.

In getting to the root of any problem, we must always look to the Bible to find the answer. It will never be found in the world. In the Bible it says, "And Adam was not the one deceived; it was the woman who was deceived and became a sinner." [2] Satan offered Eve the fruit, not Adam, because he knew that the woman is easily deceived. It's for that reason God established the husband's role as a protective covering and head over the wife. Women easily listen to and quickly believe the voice they hear in their own head. The good part about this is that we are also quick to hear God when He is speaking to us. The bad part is that we just as easily listen to the voice of the devil. On the whole I'd say that women generally hear God and respond quicker than men. A man is slower to respond to either voice. But being quick to respond is good *only* if you are responding to the right voice. To do that you must have spent enough time with the Lord in prayer and in His word *daily* to be able to discern which voice you are hearing. Is it the voice of the devil or is it the voice of the Lord?

We women must be exceptionally careful not to be duped by Satan into believing lies about ourselves. Do not listen to words such as, "You're too fat, you'll never lose weight, you can't change, you're a lost cause, you're ugly, you're old, you're a failure. Why exercise? You'll never be any differ-

[2] I Timothy 2:14 (NIV)

ent." Does that sound like the voice of God giving you
revelation for your life? Of course not! That is the voice of
the destroyer. Lies! Lies! Lies! Label it as garbage from hell
and don't listen to it. Be aware of whose voice you're
listening to. Remember from where discouragement comes
and don't let it stop you from being all that God wants you
to be. If you are seriously overweight, you are not a lost
cause. Chances are, however, that listening to the wrong
voice and believing lies about yourself is what got you into
this condition in the first place. The first set of exercises you
need to begin on immediately is in the area of the will.
Begin to say, "I *will not* believe lies about myself anymore."
I do not have to be trapped in a fat body." "I am not a lost
cause."

Ask any insurance company and they'll tell you that
overweight people have more health problems and a greater
chance of dying prematurely than those of normal weight.
God did not create you to be sick and die prematurely.
That's Satan's idea. But it's not too late for you. You will be
able to see a great difference in your entire body in just
three months of following the Seven Steps to Greater
Health.

If you need to lose weight, your metabolism *must* be
stimulated to burn calories faster than it has been. Exercise
is a must. EXERCISE IS JUST AS IMPORTANT IN
WEIGHT LOSS AS PROPER DIET IS. It develops muscle
tissue, and the more muscle tissue, the higher your metabolism. The higher your metabolism, the more calories you
burn. If you use more calories through exercise than you
consume in food, you will lose weight. Forget the gadgets,
wraps, powders, pills, vinyl suits, fad diets, reducing belts,
and all other gimmicks. You are guaranteed to put weight
back on immediately after you stop using them. You need a
way of life that is consistent and keeps your weight and
health at the optimum *all* the time.

The best way to lose weight or to control it is to eat food
the way God made it, get daily exercise, and observe all of
the other seven steps. If you go on quick-weight-loss diets
you lose water and muscle tissue and then if you gain the
weight back, you gain fat. So you end up becoming fatter

than before and as a result you will be more tired and less active. If you exercise and eat correctly, this won't happen. Eating less but better-quality food and getting more exercise are the keys. Because exercise suppresses the appetite, you end up eating less. Exercise does *not* stimulate the appetite, as some people fear. It is crucial to eat right, however, because if you eat poorly you won't have the strength you need.

I've seen people exercise like crazy for years but never change their eating habits and the results are only about half of what they desire. I've also seen many people diet and diet, and even fast and diet, and they make no lasting progress because they did not exercise. Their metabolism had practically slowed to a halt because of that excess weight, and without exercise to get it going again nothing happened.

When you exercise, you can enjoy eating more knowing that it's going to be used for energy and for fat. If you do something every day, no matter what it is, you will end up with an active life and fewer pounds.

Remember that when you exercise *muscle builds* and *fat burns*. It is always that way. A woman about fifty pounds overweight came up to me after one of the exercise classes I was teaching and said, "I don't want to exercise until I get thin because I am afraid I will firm up my fat." I chuckled over that statement until I remembered that I myself had believed the very same thing at one time. It's a real concern of many people, but let me assure you that this is *impossible* —fat and muscle are two separate things and always will be no matter how overweight you are. Muscles are always with you. They are either weak or strong. Fat is not necessarily always with you. It can come and go depending on how you treat your body. When you exercise, *muscle builds* and *fat burns*. That is why weight loss does not show as much on the scale when you first begin exercising, because the muscles are firming as the fat is fading.

If you're a chronic scale watcher, you can go crazy sitting in judgment daily on yourself as you exercise. You'll feel like you're not getting anywhere because you're killing yourself and not showing much change on the scale. Once again, get your eyes off the scales, charts, people, rates, measurements, and expectations, and get your eyes on the Lord and His ways. Be concerned with disciplining yourself to live the way you should. Do what is right and the weight will balance out without you watching it. Don't worry that you're not showing a weight loss on the scale when you begin exercising. That's because your muscles are firming up and becoming more solid. The fat will be coming off— don't you worry. Look more at whether you are starting to feel more comfortable in your clothes as opposed to what the reading is on the scale.

I can honestly say I have never met a longtime over- weight person who exercised regularly. Overweight people do not like to exercise because it requires a great effort to move all that extra weight around. Many overweight people think of themselves as inherently inactive people when in truth it is the weight that makes them that way. It's easy for a thin person to be active but it is not easy for one who is overweight. However, once you begin to move, even if it's only walking, your metabolism will begin to pick up. The more you do the more you'll feel like doing. But you *have to start somewhere* and you have to be consistent.

Attention! Attention! Repeat after me: I CANNOT HAVE HEALTHY WEIGHT LOSS AND EXPECT TO MAIN- TAIN IT WITHOUT SOME FORM OF REGULAR EXER- CISE. I want you to be convinced that if you need to lose weight and you are not exercising the whole body regularly, it isn't going to happen. Bob and Yvonne Turnbull said something wonderful in their book *Free to be Fit:* "Fat does not belong just to your abdomen, hips, buttocks, or thighs. Fat belongs to your entire body. The only way that fat is going to disappear from a specific region is if the body's calorie demand is so great that the fat is consumed as fuel." I found this to be a tremendously liberating statement and right in keeping with my quest for simplicity. You don't have to be concerned with your inner thighs, buttocks, stomach, or hips—just be concerned with exercising the whole body properly and the fat everywhere will eventually be lost.

However, if you want it all to happen quickly, you're in for a disappointment because it takes time for the body to make all the adjustments it needs to make while losing weight. Everybody responds differently. Be patient enough to keep doing what you know is right. The older we get the *less* we need to eat and the *more* we need to exercise because our metabolism slows down. The reason people gain weight as they get older is that they keep eating the same amount of food as when they were young, but they are less active.

If you are more than forty pounds overweight, check with a doctor about your health, especially about the condition of your heart. If you are okay, begin to eat food the way God made it, eliminate all the foods on the foods-to-avoid list, and begin to walk every day. That's all! Don't worry about weight loss right away. Be concerned with becoming healthy and establishing good eating habits. Faithfully observe the other seven steps. Then, after a month of good eating (or two months if you've been a junker and need to establish good health again), begin to cut down on the portions of weight producing foods, such as meat, bread, and dairy products. Remember, I said cut down—not starve. As you cut down on the portions begin to increase your physical activity. You must be doing something every day for at least twenty minutes.

Repeat after me: I MUST LEARN TO VALUE MY BODY FOR ALL THE THINGS IT CAN DO, NOT FOR HOW IT LOOKS. If your body is healthy enough to care for a home, raise children, accomplish some work each day, minister to the needs of others, remain cheerful, remind friends of their good qualities when they can't see for themselves, give of yourself to those who need you, make life more beautiful because of the special touches only you can bring, be happy with all of this. Begin to view a life of activity and regular exercise as an opportunity to build reserves of energy and to obtain good health and keep it. You are fearfully and wonderfully made. Learn to love the body God gave you. If you have mistreated it, that's not His fault. But God's mercies are great and He gives us a body that will repair and normalize and balance itself if we live the way He intended us to live. So no matter what shape you are in, there is hope for you. In fact, as I said before, you can have a whole new body in two years if you learn to live God's way and follow the Seven Steps to Greater Health. You are not a lost cause!

Forty Good Reasons to Get Up and Do It

Regular exercise will accomplish many things. Go through the following list and check the ones that matter most to you. Read the list again when you are vacillating over whether to exercise. Surely something in this list will speak to your needs.

Forty good reasons to exercise are:

1. to increase your endurance
2. to make you less susceptible to disease
3. to strengthen your heart muscles
4. to improve your complexion
5. to reduce tension and enable you to handle stress more effectively
6. to help you to lose weight and keep it off
7. to help prevent constipation
8. to lift your spirits
9. to improve your sleep
10. to clear your mind and make you more alert by stepping up the flow of blood to the brain
11. to relieve depression
12. to elevate beta-endorphic levels in your blood, which reduces pain
13. to cause your nervous system to function more efficiently
14. to increase self-esteem, confidence, and a feeling of self-worth
15. to ease your heart's work load by causing your muscles to use oxygen more efficiently
16. to relieve menopausal symptoms
17. to relieve tension headaches
18. to ease back problems by strengthening stomach muscles
19. to reduce neck and shoulder pain

20. to purify your blood
21. to aid your digestive process
22. to retard premature aging
23. to increase flexibility
24. to ease menstrual cramps
25. to reduce varicose veins
26. to relieve arthritis
27. to cut addictive cravings
28. to decrease cholesterol
29. to relieve hypertension
30. to balance your metabolism
31. to help you lose inches
32. to improve your posture and general appearance
33. to eliminate chronic fatigue
34. to give you strength
35. to reshape your body to fit more attractively into your clothes
36. to improve your circulation
37. to stimulate processes of absorption and elimination
38. to make you a more cheerful person
39. to cause your bone marrow to increase its production of red cells and increase the volume of blood
40. to help you to regulate an out-of-control appetite

For the Purpose of Godliness

There is an obvious relationship between the words "disciple" and "discipline." God calls us to be disciples and prepares us for His magnificent plans and purposes. One of the ways He does this is through discipline. A simple discipline like regular exercise helps to establish discipline in other areas of life. Physical discipline can lead the way to spiritual discipline. Each influences the other. And spiritual discipline has its end in full service of the Lord. We were created to serve a loving, caring, perfect God. It is a great calling, and we can do it best in a strong, healthy body. (Notice I didn't say a skinny body that looks great in a bikini.) The reason you need to exercise is for your health. The reason you need to discipline yourself is for the purpose of godliness.

When you are self-conscious around other people, you lose a lot of your power for ministry. If you're always nervous about how you look or what you lack, you can't be free to worry about how *other* people are feeling and what *they* need. Our insecurities are sinful because they hurt not only us, but others, too. Regular physical exercise can minimize some of our insecurities. Remember, however, that the enemy doesn't ever want you disciplined. He sees the spiritual implication of what you are doing and will try to undermine all your efforts by flooding you with temptation to fall back into old habits that are more in line with his plans. If you've been thinking to yourself, "I'm a failure because I've never done anything with my life and I don't really have a ministry," you've been listening to the wrong voice again. You need to know that you are just as important to God as any television evangelist, any entertainer, any writer or painter, any speaker or pastor.

No one ministry is better than any other. You see, we don't know the full extent of how God uses us. I've been blessed by the mere existence of certain people. They don't have to do anything for me — just seeing them and knowing that they are alive brings joy and strength to my life. You could be doing that for others, too. Don't rate yourself — God does not have a rating system. God does not critique your ministry and give you a review. You just follow hard after God and He will establish your ministry, whatever it may be. We weren't *all* meant to be missionaries to China (think how crowded it would be if we were all over there anyway!). No matter what your ministry is, being disciplined in the care of your physical body is a part of it.

In her book *Fun To Be Fit* Marie Chapian states, "You'll never have the body the Lord wants you to have without having His mind as well." This is so true. You must have *His* mind to keep you balanced, motivated, disciplined, free from pride, and consistent. As you seek to have His mind, He will speak to you about changing your way of living. When He speaks to you about something that you are doing wrong (overeating?), or not doing at all (exercising?), do not ignore Him. He calls us *all* to obedience and *obedience is healthy*. Believe me when I say you'll feel better in every way if you obey.

Be active for the purpose of godliness. God is preparing you for something good, so don't settle for anything less than what He intends. Don't underestimate your potential, for potential is in you in the name of Jesus. Give yourself totally to Him and be willing to pay the price of discipline and obedience. It's a small price to pay for the great rewards. "He who heeds discipline shows the way to Life." [3]

You Must Be Convinced

All the muscles in your body were meant to be used. In fact if you don't exercise, you leave your body to chance. You don't want anything in your life left to chance. That's not good enough. Regular exercise will help to establish healthy disciplines that will give you energy and promote peace and well-being. I want to help you make exercising a way of life and not something you struggle for. I'm not going to tell you specifically how to do certain exercises or where to buy good running shoes. There are many excellent books on those subjects. What I want this chapter to accomplish is to convince you that you need to exercise and that it must become a way of life. Each of the seven steps must become a part of your way of life.

I called my aerobics album "Exercise for Life" not only because it helps to increase the length and quality of life, but because exercise is a lifetime thing.

Some say it takes twenty-one days to establish a lifelong habit. Others say it takes ten weeks. For the purposes of this book, because there are many different elements involved in the seven steps, give yourself three months to begin to establish good habits and see a new person emerging.

Becoming healthy does not have to be miserable, painful, or even boring. You will find great enjoyment in living the way God intended you to live, and you'll be very aware of the wonderful qualities of that kind of life. You must be convinced that not one of the Seven Steps to Greater Health can be left out, including exercise. They all work together to make you healthy, youthful, attractive, and alive.

[3] Proverbs 10:17 (NIV)

Words of Truth

"Do you not know that your body is the temple
of the Holy Spirit who is in you, whom you have
from God, and you are not your own? For you
were bought at a price; therefore glorify God in
your body and in your spirit, which are God's."
I Corinthians 6:19-20 (NKJ)

"He will die for lack of discipline,
led astray by his own great folly."
Proverbs 5:23 (NIV)

"Like a city whose walls are broken down
is a man who lacks self-control."
Proverbs 25:28 (NIV)

"For a man's ways are in full view of the Lord
and He examines all His paths."
Proverbs 5:21 (NIV)

"Give me understanding and I will keep your law
and obey it with all my heart."
Psalm 119:34 (NIV)

"The Lord will perfect that which concerns me."
Psalm 138:8 (NKJ)

"And let us not grow weary while doing good,
for in due season we shall reap,
if we do not lose heart."
Galatians 6:9 (NKJ)

CHAPTER 4

Step Four: Plenty of Water

After years of research, a shocking discovery was made in 1982. The findings were published in a recent article entitled, "Researchers Find Water To Be The Perfect Drink." That's the good news. The bad news is that they spent three million dollars on their research. I didn't spend nearly that much to learn that God did not make cola, coffee, chemicalized fruit drinks, bourbon, or light beer. He made water. In fact the bodies God gave us are almost eighty-five percent water. Every cell and all tissues, fluids, and secretions of the body contain a high percentage of water. That's why you can go for several months without food, but you can only live without water for a little over a week.

If water remained in the body there would be no great need for a continual supply. But as it is, the body is constantly losing water through the ordinary processes of life. Therefore, any program for good health must take into account the body's constant need for water.

Water is involved in every single body process, including digestion, absorption, circulation, and elimination. It is the primary transporter of nutrients *through* the body and it is essential for carrying poisons out of the body—without water, none of these things could happen. With too little water these processes are very inefficient. Water helps to regulate all the body processes and body temperature.

Water makes up four-fifths of our blood, so if we want to have clean blood and stay free of disease, we must have a good supply of water coming in all the time. We need water to replace what has been lost, and water to flush out the body. Without it, certain toxic wastes will not get out.

Toxic waste products are eliminated from the body through four major organs: skin (perspiration), lungs (exhalation), kidneys (urine), and bowels (solid body wastes). These four organs must have plenty of pure water in order to do their eliminative work efficiently. When you drink plenty of water, all organs and tissues are cleansed of toxic wastes. (The average person loses about three quarts of water a day just through these natural processes.)

Next to oxygen, water is the most important element for staying alive. Nothing living can survive without it. Even the oxygen you breathe cannot be absorbed by your lungs if you don't have moisture in them. If too much water passes *from* the system it can result in dehydration. That's why it is dangerous for babies to have diarrhea for any length of time. They are small and can't afford to lose much water before a dangerously high percent of their body weight is gone.

Why Drink Water?

You may be thinking to yourself, "Everybody knows how to drink water," but let me ask you, are you drinking sixty-four ounces of fresh, pure water every day? (That's eight eight-ounce glasses.) Do you know how much you *are* drinking? Are you drinking *any* water at all? Although there is water in food, juices, and coffee, it is not the same as pure water. Pure water makes no changes when it goes into the system. It goes in, does its job, and gets out, all in the same form. Add anything else to it, like food or juice, and you've got the body sorting out the food and the water and it doesn't have exactly the same effect. That's why water is the perfect drink. Nothing else will accomplish all that it does.

How Much is Enough?

Because the body is constantly being depleted of water, you need to have a consistent supply. Average water intake should be one eight-ounce glass eight times a day. Of course, if you are tiny, or very large, or living in a desert, or doing extensive labor, or exercising, running a marathon, flying, or whatever, your need for water may be greater or less — but not a great deal in either direction.

Here is an easy way to remember to drink enough water. Drink sixteen ounces (two eight-ounce glasses) of water four times a day:

1. thirty to forty-five minutes before breakfast
2. thirty to forty-five minutes before lunch
3. thirty to forty-five minutes before dinner
4. thirty to forty-five minutes before bedtime

This way you only have to remember four times a day to drink water. How fast or slow you drink it is up to you.

Please begin by measuring the water. Drink it out of a measuring cup, or pour eight ounces into your favorite glass and see where the water line hits so you'll always be able to measure correctly. Or you can do what my husband does: he fills a plastic bottle with sixty-four ounces of water, carries it around with him, and makes sure it is gone by the end of the day. The reason for the measuring is that thirst is not an adequate indicator of your body's need for water. Because of this, doctors recommend a program of *scheduled* water intake to ensure adequate hydration. Our thirst indicators have become perverted by all the other things we drink and very few people are good judges of how much water they are getting. Pretty soon it will become second nature but you still need to check periodically to see if you are drinking enough. The basic rule is: DO NOT DRINK WATER ONE-HALF HOUR BEFORE MEALS AND FOR TWO HOURS AFTER MEALS.

We are told never to drink water *with* meals because it dilutes the digestive juices. But if you are drinking water the way I just suggested, when you sit down to a meal you will not be thirsty because your thirst has already been satisfied. You will probably only require a few sips during the meal and so you won't have to worry about that.

If you are one of those people who have difficulty swallowing water, put a few drops of fresh-squeezed lemon or orange juice in it. Remember, only a few drops. It's just to make the water palatable to you. Also, anyone who is nauseated — or experiencing morning sickness — has great difficulty drinking water. Do not force it. Try mixing equal amounts of water and juice, or just drink juice until the condition passes.

Remember that without water we cannot eliminate wastes and so people who never drink water, or drink very little, have toxic wastes accumulated in their body. This leads to dirty blood and dirty blood leads to disease. Don't let any of those things happen to you. Drink plenty of pure water to flush out your system.

When the Need Increases

Warmer weather increases your water needs, and so does physical activity. In fact, the more conditioned your body is the more water your tissues hold. Vigorous and strenuous muscle functions require still more water to carry on the work load. If drinking a lot of water is difficult for you, you will find that it gets easier as you get healthier and healthier.

Air travel also increases your water needs. Dry air combined with rapid air circulation in cabin ventilation causes large water losses. Water is lost through normal breathing and through the pores of your skin, and this contributes to the jet lag that you feel. I once read that team members of an athletic organization taking a three-and-a-half-hour flight were found to have lost as much as two pounds — or, a full quart of body water — during the flight. When I fly I make sure to compensate for this loss by drinking plenty of pure water before, during, and after the flight. I have found that it definitely does make a difference in the jet-lag experience and my skin doesn't dry out during the flight.

Carbonated drinks bloat you with gas. Sparkling mineral waters contain too much sodium. Coffee, tea, cocoa, and colas are totally dehydrating. These types of drinks should be used only on special occasions, not as a way of life, and *never* to replace water. Natural fruit juices contain water and are very good for you, but you must remember that they are a food and the body must process them differently, so don't let juices be a substitute for water.

How Pure Can You Get It?

How good is your tap water? Does it smell vaguely of bleach? What does it look like? Is it so cloudy and brown that even if you were a hippopotamus you wouldn't want to wade in it? If this is the case, call a reputable bottled-water company and begin having pure water delivered to your house. The cost of doing that will be far outweighed by what you'll save in medical bills.

You can't flush the impurities out of your system by drinking water that has more impurities than you have. If you live in an area where pure water comes out of the tap, rejoice and be thankful—there are fewer and fewer places like that in the world. It may seem unnatural to drink water from a bottle—and have to pay for it besides. But if the public water supply has become so contaminated with germs, algae, and parasites that it has to be treated with chemicals to make it drinkable at all, bottled water seems a more natural choice. Even fluoride, the miracle tooth-decay preventative, is questionable as an additive to drinking water. The point is that God did not make water that way, and man will never be able to improve upon God's ways.

Don't get me wrong, I thank God that our government chooses to treat our water with chemicals rather than allow us to have outbreaks of typhoid or cholera or whatever else could be spread by contaminated water. But it is now found that water supplies in certain areas are filled with pesticides, arsenic, asbestos, and other destructive chemicals that have been carelessly used near water supplies and have seeped into them. Pure water is not something we can take for granted anymore. This is sad but true. If we had access to pure water the way it comes from a well—fresh, clear, cool, and refreshing—there would be no need to remind people to drink water. They would do it automatically. Water like that is tasty, healing, and therapeutic. But what should be pure has been polluted—and so what should be free has to be paid for, what should be everywhere has to be searched for, what should be a regular part of our lives has to be scheduled into our day.

I grew up with well water. We had no plumbing and no running water on our farm in Wyoming. If you wanted a drink, you drew it up by hand from the pure-water well just a few feet from the house. I still remember how cool and wonderful and refreshing that water tasted. My parents retired to a small farm in central California that also has a fresh-water well. Now, of course, the water is pumped electrically into the house but that same wonderful taste is still there. It's unlike any other water—even the bottled kind.

Many people find a home water purifier to be more convenient than buying bottled water. The good ones are costly but last a long time and also purify *all* your water (bath water, wash water, etc.). I have many friends who have done this and they rave about it. They say not only do you have good drinking water, but your clothes get cleaner, your hair shinier, and there is a difference in your skin after bathing in it. I've never done that myself but have heard many positive comments about it. A purifier is something you take with you when you move. I'm not talking about the inexpensive ones that fasten onto your faucet—I'm told that they accomplish very little. I'm referring to the costly ones that are attached to your main water source. If you're ever in doubt about your water supply, you can boil the water for twenty minutes to remove much of the impurity. Do this for emergencies only, however, because although you can destroy bacteria that way, it makes for a heavier concentration of metals after some of the pure water is lost as steam.

When I began teaching the Seven Steps to Greater Health in classes, one of the first things I did was to get the ladies drinking fifty to sixty-four ounces of water every day. A few of them developed sores in their mouths, but they had been drinking tap water and had not seen the importance of buying pure bottled water as I had recommended. Now if I am teaching a class in a polluted-water area, I no longer merely suggest they drink bottled water, I make it required.

Upon switching to the pure water, the problems go away. If you end up drinking purified or distilled water be certain to eat foods high in minerals so as to replace the minerals you are not getting in your drinking water.

Water and the Skin

Water regulates body temperature by evaporating on the skin when we perspire. This evaporation cools the body. When the weather is humid, perspiration cannot evaporate, and you feel much warmer than you would in dry heat of the same temperature. The skin eliminates waste from the body continuously but especially when you are exercising and when you are sleeping. Skin is constantly breathing. In *Back to Eden,* Jethro Kloss says, "If a coat of paint or varnish were applied all over the body, a person would die almost as quickly as if a dose of poison had been given. The millions of little sweat glands are actively and constantly engaged in separating from the blood impurities which, if retained, would cause disease and death."

You can smell things like tobacco, liquor, or garlic on the skin, not because the skin has come in contact with them, but because the skin eliminates them from the body.

Body tissue is poisonous once it is dead and dead cells must be removed. When we drink plenty of pure water the poisonous wastes are flushed out of the system. The poison that comes out through the millions of pores in the skin must be removed by showering or bathing. To keep your skin and body healthy and free from a building up of toxic wastes, daily external cleansing is a must, even if it's only a two-minute shower. You may think this entirely unnecessary to mention in a health book, for surely everyone knows enough to take a bath or shower every day. However, you would be surprised at how many people think of bathing as unimportant, a luxury, or something that you do occasionally for other people's benefit. They don't realize that too infrequent bathing can lead to unhealthful conditions and disease in their own bodies.

People in Jesus' time did not bathe nearly as often as we do today. But let's face it—they didn't need to. They didn't live with the pollution, the stress, and the toxin-producing processed foods that we have today. They could probably go ten times longer without a bath as we would today and not be one-tenth as offensive.

The Dry Brush and the Loofa

The dry brush and loofa are things that many people have never heard of but which offer great benefits.

The dry brush is a brush of natural-bristles, as opposed to nylon or synthetic fibers that can damage the skin. The brush is about the size of your hand and the handle is about eighteen inches long. *Before* your bath or shower, you use the dry brush to brush every bit of skin on your body, except your face (the skin on your face should be treated more delicately, with granular cleansers, oatmeal scrub, or a soft brush). This loosens all the dead cells and body wastes that have surfaced during the night or since the last time you bathed, and then when you shower or bathe, all the impurities go down the drain. There you are with clean, clear, glowing, healthy skin.

The loofa is a long, coarse, cylindrically-shaped sponge. Even if you've never used one you may have seen them in stores and wondered what such a primitive old sponge was doing there. It looks like someone must have caught it by mistake on the end of a fishing line. The loofa is different from the dry brush in that you use it *in* the shower. After you are totally wet, you run the loofa over every bit of skin, excluding the face. It is invigorating and cleansing.

If the skin is inactive and the pores are clogged with dead cells, impurities remain in the body. This means that the other eliminative organs — including the liver, kidneys, and bowels — will have to work overtime to do the job. Can you believe that more than a pound of waste is eliminated through the skin daily? That's about one-third of all the body's impurities. In *Every Woman's Book* Paavo Airola says, "The chemical analysis of sweat shows that it has almost the same constituents as urine." Upon reading that shocking bit of information, I quickly grabbed my loofa and leaped into the shower immediately. If that doesn't convince you to bathe often and use a dry brush or loofa, I don't know what would. But in case you're not convinced yet, here are seven more great reasons to use a loofa or dry brush:

1. to remove dead cells and waste products that surface through the pores of your skin
2. to keep your pores open so your skin can breathe and do its job properly
3. to aid in the elimination process of the skin
4. to stimulate circulation
5. to improve general health
6. to make your skin more youthful by helping to avoid premature aging
7. to help you feel clean and rejuvenated.

You need to wash the dry brush and loofa every few weeks in warm soapy water and let them dry thoroughly in the sun. You will be surprised to see how much junk collects on them. These brushes are like toothbrushes — everyone should have their own.

It costs only a few dollars for a dry brush or loofa sponge and it takes only two minutes a day to use them, but it benefits the body greatly.

The Great Whirlpool Bath

Water used on the skin is healing, rejuvenating, cleansing, relaxing, soothing, quieting, and restorative. It is a natural therapeutic aid. Hot water circulating in a whirlpool bath is very relaxing and healing. Many people who don't have a swimming pool are now investing in these baths and find them wonderfully beneficial. They are as close as you can come to recreating a natural hot springs in your home. If you live under stress, have a nerve-wearing job, can't sleep at night, or are plagued with sore, aching muscles and joints, you might consider getting one for your house or yard. A word of caution: Be certain to have the whirlpool bath (or pool) fenced in completely with a gate and lock. The number of children who drown in unlocked pools is horrifying. If you can't afford a pool *and* a fence then you can't afford the pool because what you really can't afford is to have a child needlessly die in your yard. So if you're considering the price of a pool or whirlpool bath don't forget to include the price of a fence or a totally childproof and safe cover along with it. Believe me, it could be vital to your family's health.

Words of Truth

*"Long ago by God's Word the heavens existed
and the earth was formed out of water and with water."*
II Peter 3:5 (NIV)

"And if he is thirsty, give him water to drink."
Proverbs 25:21 (NKJ)

*"The poor and needy search for water, but there
is none; their tongues are parched with thirst.
But I the Lord will answer them...I will make rivers
flow on barren heights and springs within the
valleys. I will turn the desert into pools of water,
and the parched ground into springs."*
Isaiah 41:17 (NIV)

*"He makes springs pour water into the ravines....
He waters the mountains from His upper chambers."*
Psalm 104:10-13 (NIV)

"I will pour water on him who is thirsty."
Isaiah 44:3 (NKJ)

*"To him who is thirsty I will give to drink
without cost from the spring of the water of life."*
Revelation 21:6 (NIV)

*"Jesus answered, 'Everyone who drinks this water
will be thirsty again, but whoever drinks the water
I give him will never thirst. Indeed the water
I give him will become in him a spring of
water welling up to eternal life."*
John 4:13-14 (NIV)

CHAPTER 5

Step Five: Prayer and Fasting

Don't you dare skip over this chapter! This is one of the most important of the Seven Steps to Greater Health. The effects of fasting are life-giving and life-changing. Don't say, "Not me! I can't fast! I fasted once and got a headache! I've heard you can die if you skip a meal! I want to have perfect health and still be able to do my own thing. Fasting is definitely not my thing. It's weird! It's odd! It's fanatical! It's religious! It's uncomfortable! No, no, a thousand times no!"

Please calm yourself, and just hear me out. Fasting is not a torture, it is a key to a better quality of life.

To fast means to abstain from all or certain foods, traditionally in observance of a holy day. In his book *Fast Your Way to Health* J. Harold Smith describes fasting as "a turning of one's back on food as you confront the far greater need to satisfy the cravings of the inner man."

There are many things we need more than food and you will find that abstaining from all or certain foods for a period of time is a small price to pay for them. Even if you have never fasted before or think you can't, read this chapter. You may learn some wonderful new things about yourself and you might see new possibilities.

Fasting is a discipline that God designed for each one of us to bring us into a greater knowledge of Him, to release us into more fullness and power of the Holy Spirit's work in our lives, and to bring us to a point of greater health. Fasting can alter our lives in such a way that we are able to

move in new freedom, new closeness to God, and new unity
with our fellowmen. I want all those things, don't you? Of
course you do!

What the Bible Says

The kind of fasting God wants us to do is designed "to loose
the bonds of wickedness, to undo the heavy burdens, to set
the oppressed free, and break every yoke." [1] That should be
enough right there to perk your interest. Who among us
doesn't sense evil lurking around the corner of our lives?
Who wouldn't like to see the plans of the devil undermined?
Is there anyone who wouldn't like to have at least one less
burden to carry? Who has never dealt with some type of
oppression in their lives? What person doesn't need more
freedom in their inner being? This and more is waiting to
happen to you and through you. In fact, Scripture even tells
us that there are certain things that cannot happen except
through prayer and fasting.

So what are we waiting for? Why do we hesitate? I'll give
you two reasons: ignorance and fear. We are ignorant of
what the Bible says about the subject, what God wants
from us, what can be accomplished by fasting, and what all
the wonderful benefits are. We are also afraid we might die
in the night if we go to bed without dinner.

There are over eighty references to fasting in the Bible —
in the Old *and* New Testament. It is an established, proven,
practical, biblical discipline, ordained by God and practiced
by very respectable people. And yet there seems to be some
mysterious cloud of confusion around it. The mere idea of
fasting often elicits responses like "strange," "offbeat,"
"fanatical." But it should suggest words like obedience,
deliverance, wholeness, communion, discipline, and health.

If fasting was dangerous or something to fear, why would
it be mentioned throughout the Bible? Why would the
greatest people of biblical history have done it, and why
would Jesus have fasted for forty days? "After fasting forty
days and forty nights, He was hungry." [2] In fact Jesus

[1] Isaiah 58:6 (NKJ)
[2] Matthew 4:2 (NIV)

made it clear we should fast when He said, "When you fast, do not look somber as the hypocrites do."[3] Notice Jesus did not say *if* you fast, implying that maybe you *won't*, but He said *when*, assuming that you *will*.

There are many biblical examples of fasting, from Moses to David to Daniel to Hannah to Anna to Elija to Jesus Himself. I'm not going to list all of the many fasts of biblical history or even make a scriptural case for fasting because this has been dealt with so well in other books devoted to the subject. (I have listed a few of the best of these books in the appendix for those of you who want more information.) Let me just say this: *fasting is scripturally right and spiritually needed.* It is not an ancient, outdated practice but, like the Bible, it is for today.

Spiritual Discipline

Fasting is a spiritual exercise and discipline. It is a denial of self. When you deny yourself, you position the Lord as *everything* in your life, and then there is no end to the wonderful possibilities for you. Deliberately denying yourself food for a set period of time in order to give yourself more completely to prayer and closer communication with God has great rewards. Discipline always has its rewards. A physical discipline, like exercising, has physical rewards. Spiritual disciplines like fasting have spiritual rewards. It's one thing to say, "I believe in God," and do nothing. It's quite another to say, "I believe in God and desire to live the way He wants me to live," and then be obedient to all that He has commanded.

We all have a side to us that would rather smoke cigarettes than avoid lung cancer. We would rather strain our heart with many extra pounds of excess weight than curb our eating habits. We would rather miss out on a complete cleansing of our spirit and bodies than deny our tastebuds their favorite experience for a while. We get so prideful that we don't want to deny ourselves anything, but the truth is that we are much happier when we do, and so much richer when we do it all to the glory of God. In his book *God's Chosen Fast* Arthur Wallis says, "Pride and a

[3] Matthew 6:16 (NIV)

too full stomach are old bedfellows. Fasting, then, is a divine corrective to the pride of the human heart. It is a discipline of the body with a tendency to humble the soul." When you discipline yourself to do something, that means you are serious about it. Obeying the Lord and seeking a closer walk with Him through the regular discipline of prayer and fasting is worth getting serious about.

Fasting Unto the Lord

There are many religions in which fasting is regular spiritual practice. There are also many people who fast who have no religious beliefs related to fasting, but want a natural cure or cleansing for the body. We, as believers in Jesus who take seriously the written Word of God, must do our fasting unto the Lord to honor, worship, and glorify Him. It is not just a religious exercise, it is a step of obedience to God for the purpose of ministering unto Him. Fasting, then, is a personal matter between you and God — an offering to Him — and should be approached prayerfully and by the leading of the Holy Spirit. Jesus said, "But when you fast, put oil on your head and wash your face, so that it will not be obvious to men that you are fasting, but only to your Father, who is unseen; and your Father, who sees what is done in secret, will reward you."[4] This means that your fast is supposed to be observed, as much as possible, without making a big deal of it for others to notice. You don't lie about it, of course, but you don't have to be the one to bring it up.

Fasting goes hand in hand with prayer, so always fast with the intent of praying, too. Fasting is not intended to twist God's arm into getting what you want out of Him, nor is it something you do to win His approval, but it *is* a time of offering your concerns to Him. Personally, I always have a list of special burdens or needs that I bring before God with each fast. This is not to limit the Lord in what He might do, but it gives me specific points of focus when praying.

I am certain that far more is accomplished in the realm of the spirit during a fast than is ever manifested immediately

[4] Matthew 6:17-18 (NIV)

in the physical realm. I have interceded in prayer and fasting for an injured child, a friend in need of deliverance, a family member straying off the right path, the healing of someone I hardly knew, and for God's anointing of a song I was writing. To see those prayers answered was wonderful in itself, but to know that, in each case, far greater than what I asked for was being accomplished because of fasting is beyond comprehension. How great is God that He will do so much *for* us and so much *through* us, and we have to do so little ourselves. Even when you don't see the immediate direct answer to your prayer, something good and positive has transpired that you know nothing about. You can depend on that, and that is exciting! Remember that when you fast much is being accomplished in the spiritual realm even if you aren't able to pray all day long. So if you have to work during a fast day and only have time for a couple short prayers, don't feel that nothing is being accomplished —this would be far from the truth. Remember, everything you do counts, and this is no less true with fasting.

The kind of fast God wants us to have is the fast of obedience done to His glory. He wants a heart that is willing to say, "Yes, God, I'll go without food for a period if that means a child may be healed, a friend in bondage may be set free, a lost family member may be found, someone in darkness be moved into light, or that I might live in greater wisdom, peace, and power. Yes, God, a fast is a small price to pay for all that." Please be open to hear what the Lord is saying to you about fasting, for He *is* saying something. He is calling all who are able, to fast and pray. Not just a few, not just the pastors, not just the elders, not just the authors or the teachers, not just men and women over fifty-five, but all adults who acknowledge Jesus as the Son of God and abide with Him in their hearts.

Now, we don't want to be motivated to fast for selfish reasons, but there are many wonderful things that happen to our spirit and soul as a result of fasting. I have listed below a few good reasons why I have fasted in the past. I have felt the Holy Spirit prompting me for these specific reasons. Perhaps one or more of them will spark your interest and inspire you to seek the Lord more fully concerning the matter of fasting in your own life. Perhaps you will recognize in this list the very reason you need to fast and pray as soon as possible. Twenty reasons to fast are:

1. to receive divine guidance, revelation, or an answer to a specific problem
2. to hear God better and to understand more fully His will for your life
3. to weaken the power of the adversary (I find that fasting feels like getting a "holy oiling" and because of it, the world, the flesh, and the devil can't hold on to you. You slip right through their clutches into freedom.)
4. to cope with present monumental difficulties
5. to have freedom from bondage
6. to establish a position of spiritual strength and dominion
7. to be released from heavy burdens (yours or others')
8. to break through a depression
9. to invite the Lord to create in you a clean heart and renew a right spirit
10. to seek God's face and have a closer walk with Him
11. to seek the Lord when He is directing you to do something that you don't think you have the ability to do
12. to be free of evil or debilitating thoughts
13. to resist temptation
14. to be set free from everyday sins—pride, jealously, resentment, gluttony, gossiping, etc.
15. to help you when you are feeling confused
16. to help you when life seems out of control
17. to humble yourself
18. to break the lusting of the flesh after anything
19. to gain strength
20. to invite God's power to flow through you more mightily.

I don't mean to imply that the Holy Spirit will always prompt you clearly and specifically. Sometimes you will know the Lord is calling you to fast, but you will not be sure of the specific reason. It will always be easy, however, to find points of focus for prayer during fasting. There are always plenty of matters in this world worth being concerned enough about to fast and pray over them.

The spiritual side of fasting is far more significant than the physical, so do not be misled by the fact that I am writing fewer pages about the spiritual side than I have about the physical aspects. Once again, I strongly recommend that you read some of the wonderful books on fasting that I have recommended in the appendix. They are rich in scriptural insight and written by people much more qualified on the subject than I am. With that much said, let's move on to explore the physical side of fasting.

Cleansing Power

Fasting is a cleansing process from beginning to end. It cleanses your spirit, soul, mind, and body all at the same time. Physically, our bodies are constantly eliminating poisons through the lungs, skin, bowels, and kidneys. In fact, our bodies are going through miraculous processes every day, and fasting provides the most favorable conditions under which to accomplish these things. When you fast, the body is free to do the thing it does best, which is a natural self-healing and cleansing process. When you aren't filling the body with food for a period of time, all the energy that is usually used to digest, assimilate, and metabolize is now spent in purifying the body. Fasting cleans the bloodstream (remember what I have said about the importance of clean blood). When you allow the internal body to rest by fasting, a cleansing process is begun and the result is better health. Premature aging is arrested, you become more attractive, and you feel better physically, mentally, and spiritually. Every day of your fast, your spirit, soul, and body become cleaner and cleaner. Fasting is a very quick way to bring about a release of toxins from the body.

Do not think of fasting as starving your body. Think of it rather as a time of rest, rejuvenation, and cleansing — a time to stop eating to give your system a chance to renew itself. This is also a time of new cell growth even though you are not feeding the body. When you eliminate poisons and dead cells, you allow the growth of new cells. We have within us plenty of nourishment to sustain us well beyond a three-day fast. In this chapter, we are discussing only one-to three-day fasts. For longer fasts please read one of the books recommended.

Fasting eliminates poisons from the system very efficiently; when you feel a minor illness coming on, a fast can sometimes prevent its development by allowing the body to concentrate on the self-healing and cleansing process. It gives the elimination processes the opportunity to catch up on their work, and the chances are good that the reason you felt poorly in the first place was that the elimination processes couldn't keep up with all the work you were giving them. Overeating, lack of exercise, stress, eating the wrong foods, forgetting to drink water, not spending enough time in fresh air and sunshine, and not getting enough sleep allow the blood to get dirty. Your blood must be clean in order to keep disease from finding a breeding ground.

I believe that fasting is the *only* way to get rid of certain poisons. In fact, if you have taken a lot of drugs like aspirin, tranquilizers, pain killers, antibiotics, and others, fasting is a good way to rid yourself of the leftover residue that will still be floating around in your system. In the case of addiction however, seek the help of a good doctor and do not go on a self-prescribed fast. A toxic release of that magnitude could be extremely serious.

Every book I have read on fasting mentions at some point how animals naturally abstain from food for periods of time, especially when they are ill. J. Harold Smith says, "Hogs and humans are the only creatures that keep their stomachs loaded twenty-four hours a day." What a disgusting idea! I'm certain that God did not intend us to live like pigs. He intended us to live a much cleaner existence.

The cleaner you become internally the more you will desire food the way God made it and the less you will have a taste for low-quality or junk food. The same is true spiritually, too. The cleaner you become in your spirit, the less you are attracted to anything of a polluted, perverted, or unclean nature. In fasting there is cleansing power.

Physical Benefits

Even though the motive for fasting must be spiritual and the spiritual results are the most important, the physical benefits are monumental. After you have fasted for spiritual reasons and you've cleansed your body as well, you will see definite physical improvements and a more efficient mind. You will find that many small annoying physical problems begin to disappear during and after a fast. For example, if you fast regularly you will find that you are less susceptible to colds, flu, sinus problems, and various allergic reactions.

Fasting helps repair a crippled digestive tract by giving it a chance to rest from all the mistreatment it has had. Because of not eating, your stomach will begin to shrink in size, making it easier for you to control the amount of food you eat. Fasting re-educates your tastebuds, stops you from craving junk, and helps you appreciate natural foods. After a three-day fast, even the simplest foods—an apple, a baked potato, or a plain steamed vegetable—tastes like ambrosia. Don't ever underestimate the power of your tastebuds. If the fall of man came about through Adam and Eve's strong-willed tastebuds, surely this is a force to be reckoned with. But the good news is that tastebuds respond to your training. When they are disciplined sternly through fasting, they begin to act as they ought. We must always keep the body controlled by the spirit. Fasting is an effective way to do this.

Fasting helps you to lose weight (provided you don't go crazy afterward and overeat, binge, or eat unhealthful food). After each fast, you will find that more bad eating habits have been broken. I firmly believe that dieting and extreme calorie-restricted eating is much more difficult than fasting. You experience hunger all the time, and that is a painful way to live. With fasting you experience severe hunger only for the first day or two. Fasting, physical exercise, and eating food the way God made it are the keys to healthy weight loss. A low-calorie diet is torture. Fasting is not. Extreme calorie-restricted diets are unnatural. Fasting is ordained by God. Fasting helps to balance out your weight. Whether you are too thin or too heavy, regular fasting, with proper eating and exercising in between, will balance your body in every way. I must repeat that the key to achieving good healthy weight loss lies in how you eat after your regular fasts. Eating to make up for lost time is totally self-defeating.

Our bodies were not designed to be underweight *or* overweight: both conditions mean that your body is out of balance as the result of improper treatment. With proper treatment your body has to respond with natural good balance. So don't worry if you are too thin or too fat. A one- to three-day fast won't hurt you. It will rid the body of poisons, balance it out, improve your digestion and assimilation, and help you reach normal weight, no matter what weight you are to begin with. However, the time it takes for this to happen is different for each person. During a three-day fast, for example, an underweight person may find he has lost five pounds while someone overweight loses only two pounds. It seems like a cruel injustice and a sad turn of events, but if you keep fasting regularly and eat the way you're supposed to when you are not fasting, your body will balance out. An underweight person will begin to gain, and an overweight person will begin to lose.

These have been just a few of the many wonderful built-in rewards for obedience to God and for fasting to His glory. Other benefits include:

1. establishing self-control
2. curbing and eventually eliminating cravings and bad habits
3. slowing the aging process
4. adding strength (Although you may feel weak during the fast you will feel stronger than ever afterward.)
5. causing the body to consume excess fat
6. eliminating body odor and bad breath
7. giving you clear skin and bright eyes
8. eliminating chronic fatigue
9. clearing up foggy or fuzzy thinking
10. elevating self-esteem and promoting a sense of well-being

11. relieving stress, tension, and anxiety
12. saving on food bills
13. causing you to sleep better
14. ensuring that you will feel and look better.

Controlling an Out-of-Control Life

If any area of your life is controlled by anything other than God, it is out of control. It could be controlled by such things as envy, fear, isolation, depression, helplessness, eating disorders, drugs, alcohol, cigarettes, overeating, self-indulgence, lust of the flesh, television, magazines, irrational thoughts, junk food, sugar cravings, pride—the list could go on and on. Self-control is a fruit of the Spirit. Loss of control is a seed of the flesh, and Satan has a field day with it. "For a man is a slave to whatever has mastered him."[5] A life out of control can never be a life of total health. Never! You will always be driven by that which controls you.

Whatever overcomes and enslaves you, however, can come immediately under control through fasting and prayer. And you don't necessarily have to go on long fasts to do it. The wonderful news is that even a regular one-day fast each week will, bit by bit, break those bondages down and bring your life under God's control.

Sometimes we may find no particular reason for our feeling that life is out of control. When this happens, take it to the Lord in prayer and fasting immediately. You will be pleasantly surprised to see how quickly your whole physical, mental, and spiritual self can be established on a firm, calm, peaceful foundation. A fast can help you get in touch with God, your life, and difficult problems (such as your attitude toward food). The results appear so quickly that I suspect the "life-out-of-control" feeling comes straight from the devil. Through fasting and prayer, his power is totally weakened. I have experienced a complete loss of fear and depression after a one- to three-day fast.

When any area of our flesh gets out of control, fasting will

[5] II Peter 2:19 (NIV)

bring it into submission to the Spirit. During a fast, your mind has a much better chance to turn toward godly things. We must be willing to discipline ourselves in this area.

How To Fast

There are three types of fasts: absolute, partial, and total (or "normal"). In the absolute fast you have nothing to eat or drink. But I see no reason whatsoever to fast without water. If Jesus' most celebrated fast of forty days was abstention only from eating while He continued to drink water, I see no reason for you to engage in something that could be very harmful.

In the partial fast you limit your intake to juices only, or in some cases, where fasting is a medical problem, to vegetables only. (More about this later in the section "Who Should Not Fast.")

In the total fast or "normal" fast, nothing passes through the body but water. The total, or normal, fast is what I will be talking about in this book and it's the only one I recommend unless you have a medical problem and need to do a partial fast.

In fasting, as with everything else in life, you need to be organized and have some kind of plan. One of the first things you need to decide is *how long* your fast will be. It is important to do that in order to prepare your whole system. If your body and mind know that you are going on a three-day fast as opposed to a one-day, they will behave accordingly. Don't just see how long you can hold out. This is counterproductive. The fast is the Lord's. You talk it over with Him and decide beforehand the specific length, when it will start and when it will end. God is not keeping score, so you don't have to feel you're a failure if you decide to go on a three-day fast and only make it for two days. God honors what you do. Keep in mind that your body builds up and gets used to fasting just like it gets used to any other discipline. Don't use fasting as another way to be legalistic and hard on yourself, just be very clear and definite about what you believe the length of your fast should be.

In the Bible, there are examples of one-day, three-day, seven-day, ten-day and forty-day fasts. If you decide to fast longer than three days, you need to read one of the books on fasting that I have recommended to know what you are doing, or else be monitored by a doctor or nutritionist. The longer the fast, the more things you need to be aware of during it, and especially coming off of it. You need to be guided safely and I haven't the space in this book to go into that. Be sure you are knowledgeable on this subject before undertaking a fast longer than the three-day fasts I describe here.

Let me stress that fasting is not meant to be a punishment. It is a privilege. It is something to look forward to, not to dread. Remember, fasting does not mean starvation and death, it means "to abstain from." In one of his sermons on fasting, Pastor Jack Hayford said, "It is supposed to be a ministry, not a misery." So don't think of fasting as drudgery. Instead, think of all the wonderful benefits and how much you love the Lord and want to serve Him. (Before we move on, I want to stress that you will not die from a three-day fast. I don't want you to confuse the growling in your stomach with the death rattle. Believe me, they are two different things.)

Personally, I recommend a twenty-four- to thirty-six-hour fast once a week, with a three-day fast every two or three months, or as the Lord leads you. A regular discipline keeps you caught up spiritually and physically. This is not a legalistic requirement, but only a guideline.

In an article called "Guidelines for Fasting" (*Charisma Magazine,* March 1983), Derek Prince writes:

"Every Christian who decides to make fasting a part of his personal spiritual discipline would be wise to set aside one or more specific periods each week for this purpose. In this way, fasting becomes a part of regular spiritual discipline in just the same way as prayer. However, in addition to these regular weekly periods of fasting, it is likely that there will also be special occasions when the Holy Spirit calls us to fasting that is more intensive and more prolonged."

If you have never fasted, begin slowly. Try missing just one meal in the beginning, and drinking water, reading the

Word, and praying in place of the meal. Then, when you feel you are able, eliminate two meals. If you do well, the following week eliminate three meals. After you are successful on a twenty-four-hour fast one day a week for a couple months, try a thirty-six-hour fast. This means missing three meals during the day, then sleeping through the night, and eating the next morning. Work up to a three-day fast this way.

I used to believe that missing a meal or two could kill you. How far from the truth this was! Instead of dying, I began to feel more alive. When I discovered that fasting not only didn't hurt me, but helped me, the fasts became easier and easier. The more you fast, the easier it becomes. By this I mean the longer you go with your one-day-a-week fast (and three days every two months), the more poison is purged from your system, the healthier you will be, and the easier the fasts become.

Don't become a fasting maniac. It's between you and God, but it seems to me that He doesn't call people to extended fasts repeatedly in close succession. Also please don't think to yourself, "I've been eating junk and taking medicine for years, I'd better go on a forty-day fast immediately." Also do not think, "My three-day fast was so great this week, I think I'll start a ten-day fast next week." Remember, this is the Lord's fast—the one He has chosen. Begin slowly with no more than the twenty-four-hour fast at first and see how you do. Because fasting is of the Holy Spirit's leading, you can change your pattern of prayer and fasting whichever way the Spirit leads *you*. "If you are led by the Spirit, you are not under the law."[6]

Suggestions and guidelines for fasting:

1. **Decide beforehand exactly how long the fast will be.** Seek God to know specifically when to start, when to stop, and what is to be the main prayer focus.

2. **Make certain you have a good supply of pure water before you start the fast.** You need enough to last through the fast without running short.

[6] Galatians 5:18 (NIV)

3. **Drink plenty of water throughout the entire fast.** Some people recommend drinking one-half cup of water every hour. I usually can't remember to do it that often so I use the same system I described in the chapter on water (two cups upon arising, two cups before noon, two cups late in the afternoon, and two cups before bedtime). We are all individuals, so do what works best for you.

4. **Be very strict about your diet for a day or two before the fast begins.** Concentrate heavily on fresh fruits and vegetables and be strict about avoiding foods on the foods-to-avoid list. This will make the fast itself much less problematic and the benefits far greater. The body will not be clogged with overprocessed junk and the elimination system will work much more efficiently.

5. **Don't hesitate to drink a laxative herb tea when you feel the need for it.** It is very natural, mild, and beneficial. If you have a problem with constipation, drink a nice warm cup of it as the last thing you have before beginning your fast.

6. **Don't feel the fast is ruined if you happen to eat something by accident.** Just receive what you ate in the name of Jesus and return to the fast. Pastor Jack Hayford says of that, "God isn't counting calories, He's looking on your heart."

7. **Don't wander into the kitchen about four o'clock in the afternoon just to see how the pantry is doing without you.** You are setting yourself up for problems right there.

8. **Exercise lightly while fasting.** It helps you to breathe well and it generally aids the cleansing process. You should not exercise strenuously, however.

9. **Get plenty of rest.** I don't mean to suggest that you should quit working and stay home, but if you have a choice, fast on a day when your work load is lighter. Getting too few hours of sleep, working strenuously for long hours, or running all over without a moment to spare makes fasting difficult. If you're feeling especi-

ally weak or tired, or have badly mistreated your body
for sometime, go to bed during your fast or take frequent
naps.

10. **Read Isaiah 58 during every fast.** (More about this
at the end of the chapter.)

11. **Do not neglect any of the other Seven Steps to
Greater Health.** Don't forget to live peacefully; drink
plenty of water; and get light exercise, fresh air, and
sunshine, and plenty of rest while fasting.

12. **Bathe daily.** Many poisons will be coming out of your
pores and daily bathing is a necessity. Especially
important and beneficial at this time is the daily use of
a loofa or dry brush.

13. **Be very cautious about taking a sauna or a whirlpool bath while fasting.** Although they are very
therapeutic at other times, I don't recommend them
during a fast because they are too extreme. If you insist
upon doing either of these, *please* do not do it alone, but
have a non-faster in there with you. These baths are
temporarily weakening, and at certain times during the
fast there are weak periods anyway. Going into a sauna
or whirlpool that is too hot at a time when you might
be having a weak period during a fast could be dangerous. Among other things, you could get lightheaded
and faint, causing injury.

14. **Squeeze a few drops of lemon juice into your
drinking water if bad breath is a problem.** Use
fresh lemon only—no synthetics.

15. **Avoid reading cookbooks and magazines with
wonderful pictures and recipes of food.** Television
commercials can be even more dangerous. If you must
cook for others during a fast, freeze meals beforehand
(like soups) so the preparation is easier and less
tempting for you. Don't prepare your favorite dish.

16. **Avoid extremes of hot and cold** (water, baths, air
temperatures, etc.).

17. **Drink warm water while fasting if you feel
chilled (as many often do).** A good herb tea like
rosehips, chamomile, or peppermint helps a great deal.

18. **Do not take vitamins or medication while fasting, unless you absolutely must.** Pills of any kind on an empty stomach are not good for you. If it is absolutely necessary, grind the pill into a fine powder and stir it into a glass containing equal parts of water and fresh juice.

19. **Never, never, never have alcohol, tea, coffee, or soft drinks during a fast—and do not smoke!** These substances are slow killers. I certainly hope that anyone having interest enough to read a book like this would have already eliminated the terribly destructive habit of smoking. The thought of someone smoking while fasting beings horror to my heart. Please don't do it.

20. **Stand firm and resolve to continue your fast to the very best of your ability.** You will feel so much better about yourself if you do.

Symptoms of Toxic Elimination

As fasting begins to loosen the toxins in the body, there are many symptoms that give you an indication of what is going on on the inside. These signs of toxic elimination leave when the poisons are gone.

A coated tongue is a sign of toxins in the body—especially in the intestines—and often occurs during a fast. The more coated your tongue is, the more you need to be cleaned out internally. If you are bothered by a coated tongue and the bad breath that sometimes accompanies it, add a few drops of fresh squeezed lemon juice to the water you are drinking. It works as an internal cleanser and disinfectant. Check your tongue periodically anyway to see how clean or toxic you are.

Headaches are comon during fasting. They are especially common if you are new to fasting and have mistreated your body with processed food or if you regularly have caffeinic drinks like coffee, tea, or soft drinks. Headaches are a sign that the body is trying to release something impure. Any food that the body has to work hard to rid itself of instead of being able to assimilate, is an impure, headache-causing food. If your headache ever become so severe during fasting that it begins to interfere with your work and you feel you would rather take aspirin than go off the fast, do not do so on an empty stomach. I repeat: *Do not take aspirin on an empty stomach.* Instead, grind the aspirin into a fine powder (put it between two sheets of waxed paper or in a plastic bag and roll over it with a rolling pin) and stir it into about one-third cup of homemade applesauce or dissolve it into a glass of diluted fresh juice. Remember, once the poison is out of your system, the headache will go with it.

Nausea and occasionally vomiting accompany the fasts of very toxic people. Unless the vomiting is prolonged, I wouldn't be concerned about this. It is a sign that there are things in the stomach that need to come out. Think of it as a natural way for the body to rid itself of what it doesn't need. Drinking a very warm cup or two of peppermint *herbal* tea will help a great deal.

Weakness, dizziness, or lightheadedness are common. There is no reason to be alarmed by these symptoms unless they are extreme or unbearable, at which time you should simply go off the fast. Try another week or two of proper eating and following the seven steps before fasting again. "My knees are weak through fasting." [7]

Disturbed sleep, restlessness, and strange or bad dreams sometimes occur during a fast. This, once again, is because of all the poisons coming out. The good part is that you don't require as much sleep to feel rested during a fast because your body isn't exhausted trying to digest all the food you stuff into it.

Chills are common during fasting, especially when the body is ridding itself of poisons. Feeling colder happens to just about everyone. It's great in the summer to feel cool, but if you feel chilled in the winter, don't hesitate to have a cup of warm water or an herb tea (peppermint, rosehip, laxative herb, chamomile, comfrey, etc.).

Cramping in the hands, legs, and feet usually happens only during longer fasts but can happen during a one- to three-day fast, too. J. Harold Smith says, "Such cramping is the result of spasmodic contractions of the muscles working in oversensitive nerves. It can be caused by the

[7] Psalm 109:24 (NKJ)

breaking loose of long retained fecal material in the colon or the accumulation of gas from such long-held decomposing bowel content." That being the case, the healthier you are and cleaner your insides are the less that will occur. Do not be alarmed by it; it is not serious and will pass.

Cold symptoms, such as stuffy nose, clogged sinuses, or phlegm can all occur for the same reason. All of these symptoms are indicators of toxic poisons in the system and are actually signs that the body is trying to rid itself of them. They will appear less and less with each fast and eventually, if you observe all of the seven steps, they will disappear altogether.

If you experience any of these symptoms, know that it only means your fasting is even *more* necessary than you thought. It does not mean that God is telling you to forget the whole thing and have a dozen doughnuts and a pot of coffee for breakfast. In fact, what happens to you during a fast can be an indication of your health in general. The healthier you are, the easier the fast.

If any of these symptoms of toxic elimination become annoying, drink a little *fresh* fruit juice diluted with pure water. One part fresh squeezed orange juice, for example, mixed with three parts of pure water will get you through the weak periods. Drinking a vegetable broth is also excellent. You can use your imagination when making one, but the recipe I use is my own adaptation of one prescribed for me by a nutritionist. It is full of vitamins and will give you strength.

Vegetable Broth

1 onion
1 potato
2 carrots
2 stalks of celery

Peel the vegetables, cut into quarters, and add to one quart of pure water. Let the mixture simmer on the stove for one hour and then strain the solids from the broth.

When several symptoms of toxic elimination occur at one time, it is an indication that the body is going through what many nutritionists call a healing crisis. In *Nature Has a*

Remedy Dr. Bernard Jensen says, "A *healing crisis* is a process that the body goes through to eliminate accumulated toxic waste. At the time of the healing crisis we have new tissue replacing the old tissue, and this is responsible for the elimination." Again, a healing crisis is nothing to be afraid of, but something to rejoice in. During a healing crisis go to bed if you can and give yourself a rest. This will help you to get through it faster. A healing crisis can last anywhere from a couple of hours to a few days depending on how laden your body is with toxins. All these symptoms I have described are signs of a body cleansing and healing itself. Rejoice in them. They pass very quickly and the rewards are longer life and greater health.

However, if at any time these symptoms become unbearable, stop the fast and try it again at a later date. Do not feel guilty. You probably need to move slowly and pay strict attention to your eating habits. Work on the other seven steps for a few weeks to gain strength before you try fasting again. These symptoms will diminish each time you fast and eventually you will have no discomfort to speak of.

The Enema Controversy

Some doctors say that enemas are a must during a fast while others are totally against them. Those who advocate enemas while fasting say they are a must so that there won't be any decomposing putrified matter left in the bowel. Those who object to enemas say that they will irritate the bowel and wash away good bacteria necessary for normal bowel function. Let me say this. I see nothing wrong, bad, or unnatural about enemas, but I think a totally healthy body will probably never need one.

An enema is only water and does appear to be a natural form of cleansing. I have no doubt that there are many who need that. I am also certain that many people abuse the practice and take too many too often, allowing enemas to replace an activity that the body should be doing itself. Probably it depends on what condition the person is in and how toxic the bowel is. Certainly it would be better to have an enema than be totally stopped up with toxic waste. On the other hand, if you are in pretty good condition, perhaps an enema would do more harm than good. That decision is up to your own wisdom and that of your doctor or nutritionist. Be balanced.

Hunger Pangs

You will have hunger pangs while fasting, but they are more a habitual desire for certain tastes and for chewing, as opposed to any real need for nutrients. The taste buds are crying out for excitement, the stomach is growling for lack of attention, but your body already has enough food in it. If you are on a longer fast, the hunger pangs will disappear about the second or third day. Some say that the temptation to eat disappears as well, although this is not the case for all of us. Even though some of us never entirely outgrow the urge to eat, the temptation itself will change. I am no longer tempted by a chocolate candy bar, but have found myself looking longingly at an apple, papaya, avocado, or baked potato. If you have been on a calorie-restricted diet or have been starving yourself for any reason before beginning the fast, you are going to have a lot of trouble fasting. You must be eating sensibly, caringly, and with wisdom and discipline before you begin fasting. Starving yourself and then fasting is tantamount to an eating disorder and you are in for serious problems. Don't ever do that.

Every time you feel hunger pangs, drink some water and say a prayer. If that doesn't help, try warm water with lemon in it. If the hunger pangs are interfering with your work or sleep, have a glass of *herb* tea or vegetable broth. As you become accustomed to fasting, the problems that arise in the beginning will disappear.

Pay attention to any very strong and persistent cravings you have while fasting. They can be signs of a particular food with which you have overloaded your body and possibly you have developed an *allergy* to it. On my first seven-day fast under a nutritional doctor's direction, I had an almost unbearable craving for bread or toast. It was then discovered that I had an allergy to wheat. My particular allergy symptoms are extreme weakness, fatigue, weight gain, and excess phlegm. When I eliminated wheat from my diet all the allergy symptoms went away. I now eat wheat infrequently and have no problem. If I begin eating too much wheat at any time, all the symptoms return. I have discovered that if I eat homemade bread made with grains that I have ground into flour in my grinder, I have no problem. My nutritionist told me that the reason for this is that for three days after grinding, a grain remains pure and fresh. After three days a certain chemical change begins to happen which produces the irritant that can cause an allergic reaction. Once again I saw how eating pure food the way God made it, or as close as possible to the way He made it, is absolutely the most beneficial.

I am not certain how reliable craving is as an indication of allergy but it certainly is an indication that you are eating too much of a certain kind of food.

Examples of Short Fasts

A twenty-four-hour fast:

1. Stop eating after dinner on Monday night at six.
2. Eat nothing and drink only water all day Tuesday.
3. After six o'clock on Tuesday night eat a fruit salad, or a vegetable salad, or a baked potato and a steamed vegetable. If you do have something more, like meat or cheese, go very, very lightly.

Slightly longer fast:

1. Stop eating after lunch on Monday at noon.
2. Eat nothing and drink only water for the remainder of Monday and all day Tuesday.
3. For dinner on Tuesday evening at five or six o'clock, eat a fruit salad, or a vegetable salad, or a steamed vegetable and baked potato.

A thirty-six-hour fast:

1. Stop eating after dinner on Monday night at six.
2. Eat nothing, and drink only water all day Tuesday and Tuesday night.
3. On Wednesday morning break the fast with a raw or steamed apple and a papaya. Eat a lunch consisting of

a raw vegetable salad and/or a steamed vegetable and a baked potato.

A *three-day fast:*

1. Stop eating after dinner on Monday night at six.
2. Eat nothing and drink only water all day Tuesday, Wednesday, and Thursday.
3. Break the fast either Thursday evening or Friday morning with a raw apple or homemade applesauce plus an orange or a papaya. Nothing more.
4. For lunch on Friday have something like a small, fresh raw vegetable salad or a baked potato with plain yogurt on top and a steamed vegetable (like broccoli or carrots).

How to Resist When Temptation Comes

Fasting can be difficult insofar as eating with other people has become our favorite social activity. There is great warmth and enjoyment in eating a meal with friends you love, and limiting that is hard. However, you don't have to be a total hermit. A pastor and his wife, who are very close friends, invited us for dinner. The wife fixed a wonderful meal and as we all sat down together we discovered that she was fasting. She explained that the Lord called her to an extended fast after we had set the date for this dinner and she didn't want to miss the opportunity to be together. As it turned out, the evening was still perfectly enjoyable, and the fact that she was fasting did not affect anything. I admired her commitment. Her joy was infectious and it was evident that she did not feel deprived. Not everyone is that strong — I don't know if I would be — but it *is* possible to be with people and continue fasting. They will hardly notice if the conversation and fellowship is rich and vital, and you will survive it well if you keep in mind the joy that is set before you.

Some fasts are easier than others, but there are times when fasting is a constant struggle and the hunger never goes away. These difficult fasts may come as a result of some kind of bodily abuse prior to fasting. This bodily abuse can be anything from eating the wrong foods to getting no physical exercise, not enough sleep, or experiencing a great deal of stress. During these difficult fasts, I believe it is well worth your while to stick it out to the best of your ability. The following list suggests things to read, say, think, and do when the going gets rough. All of these have helped me in the past and should help you, too.

What to tell yourself when you are tempted to eat:

1. I am fasting out of obedience to the Lord.
2. I am fasting because there are yokes of bondage that need to be broken in my life and in the lives of others.
3. I am fasting because I want more of God's power working in my life.
4. The special concerns I am praying about during this fast make it well worth continuing.
5. The physical cleansing, healing, and rejuvenating that is accomplished during fasting are well worth a short time of denial.
6. At this moment there are greater things that need to be accomplished in my life than eating.
7. Eating food right now won't be as satisfying as finishing the fast.
8. "I can do all things through Christ who strengthens me." [8]

Lies to reject when you are tempted to eat:

1. "This is more trouble than it's worth."
2. "The only thing this fast is doing is making me miserable."
3. "My headache and weakness must be a sign from God that I should break the fast."
4. "Nobody else is torturing themselves like this."
5. "Nobody knows I was fasting so nobody will know that I broke it."
6. "I do all the other seven steps well. I can leave out just this one."
7. "It must be that some are called to fast and some are not."
8. "This isn't accomplishing anything; I might as well forget it."

[8] Philippians 4:13 (NKJ)

What to do when you are tempted to eat:

1. Get out of the kitchen as quickly as you can.
2. Get into the Word of God (especially Isaiah 58).
3. Drink hot water with lemon, herb tea, or vegetable broth.
4. Fix your mind on a project that interests you (do not study for your gourmet-cooking class).
5. Lie down and take a nap.
6. Go outside for a walk.
7. Start cleaning out a closet.
8. If all else fails, take off all your clothes and go look at your hips in a mirror. This is very effective in most cases.

How to Come Off a Fast

Repeat after me: HOW YOU BREAK A FAST IS JUST AS IMPORTANT AS THE FAST ITSELF. One more time, let's say it together: THE WAY YOU COME OFF OF A FAST IS JUST AS IMPORTANT AS THE FAST ITSELF. If you are going to come off of a fast by eating too much and eating the wrong kind of food, then it makes no sense to fast. You must come off a fast slowly and with control, not desperately and with the speed of lightning. The longer the fast, the more slowly and carefully you should come off of it.

For the most part, you will feel that you *want* to eat with more wisdom and control after a fast than you did before. There are three rules to remember concerning this. First: DO NOT AT ANY TIME OVEREAT WHEN COMING OFF OF A FAST. The most serious mistake you can make when fasting is to eat too much afterward. Unfortunately, that is the most common mistake, too. Always remember that your stomach will shrink during a fast and so you will not need as much food as you have been used to eating. Keep that in mind when putting food on your plate. Even though your stomach shrinks, your eyes might become larger — don't let your eyes get bigger than your stomach when it comes to food. That can end up being very painful. Breaking the fast is actually when you have to exert the most self-control. Maintain a calmness, a control, and a slow pace when approaching food.

Second: ALWAYS BREAK THE FAST WITH A RAW OR LIGHTLY STEAMED FRUIT OR VEGETABLE. *Never* break a fast with meat, poultry, milk, or cheese— let at least a meal or two go by without them. *Never, never, never* break a fast with junk food—the consequences would be horrible. After a fast, the body reacts strongly to every morsel of food. If the food is good, the reaction is good. If the food is bad, the reaction is bad. You can also break a fast with a glass of fresh squeezed vegetable or fruit juice. Do not under any circumstances use something canned or processed in any way. When you come off a fast your taste buds are appreciative of anything. Use that opportunity to give them the purest and cleanest food available. Stay away from any refined foods or seasonings for as long as you possibly can. Begin with an orange, apple, papaya, or watermelon. Homemade applesauce is also great.

Homemade Applesauce

1. Peel an apple or two and cut them into small chunks.
2. Steam the fruit in metal steamer until a fork slides easily into one of the chunks.
3. Put the fruit in a blender, add one-half to three-quarters of a cup of the water from the steamer, and blend.

(After a fast eat it plain just as it is. Later, when you want applesauce for breakfast, add a pinch of cinnamon and a squirt of honey and blend together.)

I overate after a three-day fast only once—once is all it takes to teach you not to do it again. Even though I did it on healthful food, it made me very sick. I felt so good while I was on the fast and so bad after I overate. It was a very dumb thing to do because I knew better, but I thought that after a short fast I could get away with it. I can hardly imagine how bad it would feel after a fast of any great length.

The third rule is: BREAK THE FAST WITH NO MORE THAN THREE DIFFERENT FOODS AT ONCE. For example, a three-day fast that is broken with fruit should include no more than three types, such as a combination of apple, papaya and watermelon. Just one would be fine, but

no more than three. It is too much for your system. If you
are beginning with vegetables, just have a light salad with
red-leaf lettuce, chopped avocado, and tomato or grated
carrots. Or steam some broccoli and carrots, along with a
baked potato. Believe me, after a three-day fast, this tastes
like a wonderful meal. Even when you do begin to add meat
and grains, keep it simple. Just three things. For example:
Roast turkey breast, brown or wild rice, and steamed
carrots is a good, clean, uncomplicated healthful meal.
(Just make sure that fifty percent of the meal is the carrot
dish, twenty-five percent is turkey, and twenty-five percent
is rice.) You will be amazed at how keeping your meals
completely simple after a fast really makes a difference.
You will, in fact, prefer the clean fresh tastes of simple
natural foods the way God made them. It is likely, too, your
taste will become very sensitive to chemical additives, or
unnatural ingredients in your food. Remember to continue
drinking six to eight glasses of pure water a day even after
the fast. Do not add salt, pepper, or other spices to your
food. Hold off as long as you can — forever if possible. Eat
slowly and chew thoroughly to help break down the food
properly.

High Expectations

There are all kinds of wonderful things that you can expect
to happen to you after you've been on a regular fasting
schedule for a month or two. First of all you will feel better,
stronger, and have more energy. Your skin will be clearer,
smoother, and healthier in color. Your eyes will become
bright and sparkling. You will find yourself looking and
feeling younger with each fast. (Each of the seven steps
slows down the aging process.)

Although you may experience dizziness during a fast —
especially if you stand up too quickly — after the fast your
mind will be clearer than it was before. If you are following
all the other seven steps as well, you will lose weight. The
only reason you might not lose weight during a longer fast
of three to ten days is that your body might be out of
balance and unable to respond normally. It will take longer

for you but you will eventually balance out. Don't give up.

Your taste buds will become re-educated and you will begin to have an appreciation for food the way God made it. You will begin to lose your taste for highly processed junk food and desire fresh fruit, vegetables, whole grains, and nuts. Even if you never lose the taste for a certain thing, you *will* lose the taste for what it does to you. There are certain sweet desserts that I still love, but what I love *more* is not being sick.

Menstruation will become more regular, lighter, painless, and less problematic due to regular fasting and a cleaner system. Be aware that in a fast of three days or more, your period may come a day or two later than usual. It may also be lighter and shorter. I've always had difficult, painful, long, heavy periods until I began fasting. They are now light, painless, and last four to five days. This is a wonderful benefit for many women.

Body odor will disappear. Your mouth will taste good, your breath will smell fresh, your skin will smell clean, and any other body odors you are troubled with will decrease with each fast and won't be there at all when you are totally clean.

Your outlook on life will change through fasting. You'd be surprised how burdensome it is to carry around toxic waste and how light and worry-free your attitude will be when you are cleaned out and healthy.

You will have more free time. I was shocked to discover how much time I actually spent in the kitchen every day. We fast at our house for twenty-four hours once a week, and on that day I have four to six extra hours. Figuring the time it takes to prepare the meal, set the table, clear the table, wash the dishes, and take out the trash, there is really a lot of time to be gained by not eating. Even eating out takes a good amount of time. On fast days I do quick simple meals for the children. I freeze ahead homemade soups and breads and just defrost, heat, and serve. The children love it and I spend only a short time in the kitchen. If you must cook for family members not fasting with you, don't make it hard on yourself. Plan to serve enjoyable meals that are simple to prepare. A fast is not the time to prepare your gourmet delights unless you are one who is not at all tempted.

These are only a few of the things you can expect to see happen in your life as a result of fasting. You can certainly afford to have high expectations.

Who Should Not Fast

There are those who will be unable to fast for medical reasons. "Let not him who does not eat judge him who eats." [9]

Pregnant women and nursing mothers should not fast at all. You don't want to unload your toxins on an unborn or newborn child. It is not worth the risk. Wait four to six months after having a baby before fasting. Give your body a chance to get itself back together, for the hormones to normalize, for any healing to be complete. Don't rush your recovery in any way. Give yourself a rest. Then begin slowly and work up to where you were before. If you begin anything too soon — a weight-loss program, exercise, or fasting — you can create problems for yourself that might take a year or more to recover from. Always be sensitive to your own body. Even if after six months you still don't feel up to any of these things, don't rush yourself.

Once your rest and recovery time has passed, you might find that a fast is just what you need to set you straight again. That's what happened to me after my second baby, when my recovery and weight loss were totally painless and problem-free. I started with a twenty-four-hour fast one day a week when the baby was six months old, and then progressed to a thirty-six-hour fast once a week. When Amanda was nine months old I went on a three-day fast and I can say wholeheartedly that that was a turning point for me. After that fast, I was a new person spiritually and physically. I lost my tired look, I felt stronger, I looked better than I had in over a year, my mind was clear, and I lost the "baby blues" that I had experienced after the baby was born. I'm convinced that that fast cleansed me of all

[9] Romans 14:3 (NKJ)

the medication I took for the cesarean delivery and afterward for pain. The one-day-a-week fast is a good maintenance program, but for real release of poisons, a three-day fast is better.

Anyone with a serious illness, such as diabetes, liver or kidney disease, tuberculosis, hypoglycemia, or heart problems, should not fast; nor should anyone *extremely* underweight. You must enjoy a certain degree of good health to fast, and then when you do fast your health continues to improve. Fasting releases toxins in the system that will be too stressful for someone already weakened by a disease. While it is true that fasting can help those with minor illnesses, someone who is very ill should not fast unless under the total care of a good doctor who prescribes such treatment.

For those who do have medical problems and have expressed a spiritual desire to fast, I suggest you ask your doctor if one day a week you may eat only fruits and vegetables. Quite often this is no problem whatsoever, but you need to know for certain that it would not be harmful. My seven-year-old son calls that a "vegetable-and-fruit fast." Every so often when we are fasting, he will go on that for a day and we've seen it do great things for him. In such a short time, his little brown eyes become very clear and bright, he becomes extremely cheerful, and he seems unusually peaceful. By all means, if you are physically unable for any reason to go on a regular fast, a partial fast of fruits and vegetables is certainly acceptable. The Lord most certainly honors that as a fast to His glory.

Doctors disagree on the advisability of fasting. There seems to be two extreme camps. Many have never done it and know nothing about it, or have seen the practice abused and are firmly opposed to it. On the other hand, a lot of doctors know of its value, have experienced it personally, and highly recommend it. If you trust yourself to a doctor for medical care, you must also trust his advice as far as fasting. In this case it is a matter between you, God, and your doctor.

The Road to Good Health

God gives us many wonderful keys to use here on earth —
keys like reading and speaking the Word, praise, prayer,
faith, and also fasting. Don't let your life be locked up
because you are not using your keys. Fasting is a key to
total health in every part of your being.

Fasting is not the easiest of disciplines, I realize, but it's
certainly not the hardest either. It's easier than you think.
Quite frankly, if you are living to satisfy your flesh and are
not willing to see what God's ways are and abide by them,
you will have to face the consequences. The greater the
perversion of His ways, the greater the consequences. You
need only look around you to see this. Catering to your
physical appetite or lusts will lead to problems of some sort,
and you will end up paying a price somewhere in your body
or mind. We *all* have to come to terms with God and His
ways before we can be healthy.

Assuming that you do not have a serious disease, let's
talk about achieving and maintaining good health, and
what part fasting plays in this. All members of the animal
kingdom living in a natural environment know instinctive-
ly how to heal themselves through fasting. You will find at
times — for example, when you have a cold — that the best
thing to do is to go to bed and fast for one to three days. You
may find the cold will reach its peak and dissipate in far
less time it would otherwise take. In fact, if you have
frequent colds or "bugs," fasting is your answer.

Fasting slows down the clock when it comes to aging.
Think of it in these terms, premature aging is actually a
latent disease. It is an unhealthy condition of the body.
Experts claim that fasting will add years to your life. I
believe it, and those years will be filled with vitality and
life!

People are having heart attacks and strokes at a younger
age than they use to. Poor eating, lack of exercise, and
deadly habits pav the way. Doctors usually can't find a
clogged or blocked artery until it is serious. If you are
worried about high cholesterol, try fasting to clear out those
arteries.

Constipation creates many problems. Many problems create constipation. Constipation is caused by stress and a poor diet, and fasting can relieve the results of both much better than medicine.

Weight loss is much healthier when regular fasting is a part of the program. Most people find fasting easier than a highly restrictive diet because there are no choices to make. In restrictive dieting you have to constantly decide what you will eat and how much, whereas in fasting, you do not even have to think about food.

It is becoming more and more frequent that bodies and minds are breaking down under the stresses that we subject them to. We must begin to look at illness not as a failure, but as a sign that something is out of balance. God is a god of balance. His ways are life-balancing. He has provided fasting as a way to total rejuvenation of the mind, body, and spirit.

The thing that bothered me most about being pregnant was neither morning sickness, nor labor pains, but the fact that I could not fast. I missed the especially close time I share with the Father when I fast and pray. I missed the light, fresh, renewed cleanness in spirit and body that I experience each time. I missed the sense of strength and good health. Fasting is not a cure-all, but it is one of God's ways of healing. Don't be afraid of it. Instead, fear over-weight, high blood pressure, heart failure, poor circulation, chronic fatigue, and constant illness. God designed fasting. It is in His Word. Learn of it.

God's Chosen Fast

In the Bible, God talks about the kind of fasting He desires in the fifty-eighth chapter of the Book of Isaiah. He describes the kind of fast He had chosen, what fasting is intended to accomplish, and what the promise is for those of us who fast. This chapter is powerful, and so important for everyone that I am including half of it here. *Please read it every time you fast,* or better yet, read it from your own Bible, in your favorite translation. God will speak to you through it. You will be reminded of why you are fasting: to "loose the chains of injustice," "set the oppressed free," and to "break every yoke." [10] It will also serve as a reminder of what you should do: "share your food with the hungry," "provide the poor wanderer with shelter," and "not turn away from your own flesh and blood." [11] And He tells you of your rewards: "your light will break forth like the dawn and your healing will quickly appear" and "the glory of the Lord will be your rear guard. Then you will call and the Lord will answer." [12] And ultimately you are assured that "you will find your joy in the Lord." [13] Read Isaiah 58 every time you fast, and ask the Lord to speak to your heart about what it all means. It's very rich with purposes, promises, and truth.

Isaiah 58:6-14 (NIV)

"Is not this the kind of fasting I have chosen:
to loose the chains of injustice
   and untie the cords of the yoke,
to set the oppressed free
   and break every yoke?
Is it not to share your food with the hungry
   and to provide the poor wanderer with shelter,
when you see the naked, to clothe him,
   and not to turn away from your own flesh and blood?
Then your light will break forth like the dawn,
   and your healing will quickly appear;
then your righteousness will go before you,
   and the glory of the Lord will be your rear guard.
Then you will call, and the Lord will answer;
   you will cry for help, and He will say: Here am I.

If you do away with the yoke of oppression,
   with the pointing finger and malicious talk,
and if you spend yourselves on behalf of the hungry
   and satisfy the needs of the oppressed,
then your light will rise in the darkness,
   and your night will become like the noonday.

[10] Isaiah 58:6 (NIV)
[11] Isaiah 58:7 (NIV)
[12] Isaiah 58:8-9 (NIV)
[13] Isaiah 58:14 (NIV)

The Lord will guide you always;
  He will satisfy your needs in a sun-scorched land
  and will strengthen your frame.
You will be like a well-watered garden,
  like a spring whose waters never fail.
Your people will rebuild the ancient ruins
  and will raise up the age-old foundations;
you will be called Repairer of Broken Walls,
  Restorer of Streets with Dwellings.

If you keep your feet from breaking the Sabbath
  and from doing as you please on my holy day,
if you call the Sabbath a delight
  and the Lord's holy day honorable,
and if you honor it by not going your own way
  and not doing as you please or speaking idle words,
then you will find your joy in the Lord,
  and I will cause you to ride on the heights of the land
  and to feast on the inheritance of your father Jacob."
The mouth of the Lord has spoken.

Words of Truth

"Even now," declares the Lord, "return to me with all your heart, with fasting and weeping and mourning."
Joel 2:12 (NIV)

"So we fasted and petitioned our God about this, and He answered our prayer."
Ezra 8:23 (NIV)

"The fear of the Lord is the beginning of knowledge, but fools despise wisdom and discipline."
Proverbs 1:7 (NIV)

"Everyone who has this hope in him purifies himself, just as he is pure."
I John 3:3 (NIV)

"So He said to them, 'This kind can come out by nothing but prayer and fasting.'"
Mark 9:29 (NKJ)

"I proclaimed a fast, so that we might humble ourselves before our God and ask Him for a safe journey for us and our children, with all our possessions."
Ezra 8:21 (NIV)

"For the grace of God that brings salvation has appeared to all men. It teaches us to say 'No' to ungodliness and worldly passions, and to live self-controlled, upright and godly lives in this present age, while we wait for the blessed hope — the glorious appearing of our great God and Savior, Jesus Christ."
Titus 2:11-13 (NIV)

CHAPTER 6

Step Six: Fresh Air and Sunshine

Darkness brings death; light brings life. This is true whether you're talking about the spiritual realm or the physical side of things. Unfortunately, it's a concept that, as a whole, we seem all too eager to ignore.

Over the last few decades we have increasingly left natural light and fresh air out of our lives. Man now constructs buildings with no windows at all. Already many of our schools have classrooms with no windows and our children are studying in artificial light and artificial ventilation. Research indicates a lower level of academic performance among children who must learn in these conditions. We now have hospitals where the sick are supposed to get well with no fresh air and sunlight whatsoever. There are office buildings where people work all day under artificial light breathing artificial air and go home at night feeling totally drained and irritable. The windows we do have are covered with blinds, shades, shutters, curtains, and drapes that many people keep closed during the day as well as at night because of fear, lack of privacy, ignorance, or better television viewing. We are crawling into dark man-made holes and wondering why we don't feel up to par.

The only explanation I can find for this trend is that man, left to his own devices, will shut God's wonderful natural ways out of his life, even as he tries to "improve" on them. But once again, man's ways can never be better than God's ways. You can have everything—the best food, water, plenty of exercise—but without enough fresh air and sunshine you will not have total health.

Light Up Your Life

What about you? How do you live? Do you live in a dark house? Do you keep the shades drawn all the time? Do you work in a building with no windows? Are you awake all night and sleepy all day? Do you spend time daily in the fresh air and sunlight? If not, then come out of the darkness into the light because you are not living the way God intended you to live. You are closing off one important aspect of your life. A bit of fresh air and sunshine every day is healing and rejuvenating for every part of your body. We were not created to live in dark holes. In fact, we were made to be outside most of the time, with homes to provide shelter, protection, and security. I'm talking about opening up your windows to fresh air and sunlight, and spending some time each day outdoors. I'm talking about letting fresh air and sunlight become a regular part of your life.

Sunshine is Medicine

Sunlight is a powerful healer, tonic, germ killer, remedial agent, and relaxer, especially when it is used in conjunction with the other seven steps. When you spend time in the fresh air and sunshine, your body drinks in their life-giving elements. Scientists are now discovering a great connection between light and health. They have found that natural light has a very significant effect on our immune system. Light is already being used for treating various diseases of the blood and skin, and for curing certain kinds of depression and nervous disorders. The value of sunlight for the sick has been demonstrated by hospital experience. They are finding a larger percentage of recoveries in rooms having abundant sunlight, and especially those that allow fresh air to circulate.

When the sun shines on the skin, the nerve endings absorb energy and send it throughout the entire body. This calms the nerves. We've all experienced how a few hours spent playing at the beach or working in the garden can make you feel like taking a nap. Another reason for this is that when the sun hits your skin it manufactures vitamin D in your body and then works as a great natural aid to calcium absorption. Calcium soothes the nervous system — this is why anyone suffering from insomnia or sleeplessness would greatly benefit from twenty to sixty minutes out in the fresh air and sunlight daily. Sunlight is one of the greatest sleep inducers, *especially* when you combine it with any form of physical exercise. If you were to spend an hour out in the sun gardening every day, your entire being would show favorable changes. You always sleep better at night when you spend enough time in fresh air and sunshine during the day.

The opposite is also true. If you are feeling fatigued or sluggish, just stepping outside for a walk in the fresh air and sunshine will *energize* you. That's because *all* the natural ways of God are *balancers*. They balance out the body and make it whole.

The rays of the sun also have germ-killing properties. Wounds exposed to air and sun will heal more quickly than those that aren't. However, exposing wounds to intense, prolonged, direct sunlight will sometimes cause the wounded skin to turn brown. That's why bandage companies are now making bandages that breathe. They protect the wound while allowing fresh and natural air, so crucial for healing, to touch it.

The healthier you are, the more you will be attracted to fresh air and sunshine and being outdoors. The healthier you become, the more you will find yourself opening windows, forgetting to put up your drapes, and desiring to be in homes, schools, health clubs, banks, and office buildings that have an abundance of natural light in them. In fact, you will begin to see anything else as dreary.

Light and Mental Health

It is definitely true that a person thinks differently when he sits in a room without windows, natural light, or ventilation than he does when he sits outdoors surrounded by the beauty of nature. We all notice that people, including ourselves, feel and act more depressed or irritable when exposed to too many consecutive days of cloudy, rainy, or foggy weather than they do when the days are bright, clear, and sunny. The wonderful surroundings of nature combined with fresh air and sunlight act to soothe and refresh the mind.

In the April 1982 issue of *Psychology Today* there was an article by science writer Hal Hallman that talked about new discoveries concerning the connections between light and health. He cited a case of severe depression being treated by psychiatrist Alfred J. Lewy. In this particular case the problem was due to lack of exposure to sunlight. The article reported that: "all aspects of our health— mental, emotional, as well as physical—are indeed effected by the intensity of light to which we are exposed"; "light is being used to treat various diseases of the blood, skin, and other parts of the body"; "light can also alleviate certain kinds of depression, jet lag, and sleep disorders." If all these wonderful things can happen for those who have severe problems, think what fresh air and sunshine can do for you and me who suffer from minor irritations, like frequent colds (fresh air and sunshine are germicidal), insomnia (sunshine soothes frayed nerves), sluggishness (sunshine is a healthful stimulant), or depression (sunshine is an anti-depressant).

There is a gland in the brain that can be reached by light traveling through the eyes. The release of hormones is regulated by this gland. Our hormone system responds to light, and hormones control many of our bodily functions and even affect our mental stability. If you notice seasonal changes in your mood—for example, if you are prone to depression in winter and feel great in the spring, or tend to feel "down" on rainy days and "up" on sunny days—this could be a sign that you need *more* exposure to fresh air and sunlight on a regular basis. For mental as well as physical health, frequent exposure to fresh air and sunshine needs to become a part of your way of life.

Artificial Lighting

Man can never improve upon what God has made—this includes light. We now spend a lot of time in artificial light, which differs drastically from sunlight in both character and intensity. In fact, studies have found that fluorescent lighting is depleting, depressing, and destroys certain vitamins. If you are living or working in fluorescent lighting, make an effort to see what you can do to change these conditions. If regular lighting or natural-lighting sources can't be installed then see about changing locations. If you can't change the lighting and you can't leave that building, then make especially certain that you are getting plenty of fresh air and sunshine outdoors. Your body is being depleted if you are forced to spend much time in such an unhealthful condition.

Seek out natural lighting whenever possible. If you have a choice, choose light over darkness, choose natural light over man-made light, and choose standard lighting over fluorescent lighting. It will add up to a big difference in your health.

For example, if you have work to do (it could be anything from writing a book to shelling peas) do it where you can get the most fresh air and natural light. If you're writing a letter, sit next to an open window. If you are sewing a button on a shirt, sit out on your patio or front steps. Eat outside whenever you can, and choose airy, sunny restaurants as opposed to those so dark an owl would have trouble finding his way to the table. When choosing light, choose it as natural as you can get it.

Life Comes From the Sun

Fresh air and sunshine are life giving and that's what we're after. We want more life, not sickness and a daily dying in our physical bodies. Without fresh air and light, we, along with all forms of life, would die.

There are hidden life-promoting qualities in food that is grown and ripened in the sun. Many of these wonderful healing properties can be obtained just by eating sun-ripened fruits and vegetables. The tremendous restorative powers in such foods serve to bring about great strength in the body. Because food grown in the sun is absolutely essential for life, try to see that fifty percent of each meal includes fresh fruits and/or vegetables. If you have sun on

the outside and sun-grown foods on the inside, you will
have wonderful, glowing health.

In plants the sun produces chlorophyll, which is a
wonderful healer and cleanser in the human system. In
fact, it has been said that chlorophyll is "life from the sun."
That is why you'll hear so many nutritionists and health-
minded doctors recommending steamed beet tops, chard,
spinach, parsley, endive, or red-leaf lettuce in your diet. All
that natural chlorophyll is healing and cleansing.

There was a period a few years back when my husband
and I had time to tend a garden. We dug up a large portion
of our backyard, brought in some fertile soil, planted and
grew all our own vegetables. It was greatly invigorating to
work outdoors in this garden every day and it was
wonderful therapy for the whole family. We had much
success and the garden yielded huge amounts of beautiful
sun-kissed vegetables. Whatever we wanted for lunch or
dinner, we went out and picked from our garden just prior to
preparing it.

Not only was gardening a fulfilling experience for all of
us, there were incredible physical benefits besides. I noticed
that my fingernails were the strongest and the longest they
had ever been; my skin was exceptionally clear and healthy
in color; my hair became thicker and had an exceptional
sheen; I slept more deeply and soundly at night than I had
ever slept before and I *never* woke up tired; I felt strong and
energetic *all* the time; and people constantly commented on
how rested and healthy I looked.

The results I experienced were also noticeable in all of the
other members of my family. None of us were ever tired, let
alone sick, during that time. Of course we were following all
the Seven Steps to Greater Health all the while. There was
such a difference that I knew we were on to something:
eating fresh fruits and vegetables, *grown* and *ripened* in the
sun and picked just before eating, had miraculous healing
and rejuvenating effects. And this is the way God has
always intended us to eat.

Later, when that period of our lives ended and it came
time for us to travel, keeping a garden that required daily
care became impossible. But I found within five miles of our

home a wonderful fresh-fruit-and-vegetable stand that, between April and November, sold fresh fruit and vegetables picked that day. It's not quite as good as having your own garden, but it's certainly worth the trouble to get the benefits of fresh foods grown and ripened in the sun. Search and see if there is not a place like that near you as an alternative to buying foods that have been picked prematurely and ripened artificially.

Physically Active in the Great Outdoors

As you become healthier and healthier (living peacefully, eating food the way God made it, exercising regularly, drinking plenty of water, fasting and praying, and getting good rest), the greater your desire to be outside in the fresh air and sunshine. If, on top of that, you can engage in some kind of physical activity while you're outside, it is one of the best things you can do for yourself.

It is not healthful to live a sedentary life totally indoors. We were never made to live like that, and we will suffer in our bodies if we continue to do so. I've seen people who were sickly and suffering from insomnia and nervous disorders become new people when they took on a program of physical activity in the great outdoors. They had new color, and I'm not speaking just cosmetically, for this happened in the autumn when they could not have gotten a tan. They slept better at night, their mental attitude improved, and they became new people. Swimming, tennis, hiking, jogging, walking, weeding the flower beds, mowing the lawn, fixing a broken screen, washing the windows, waxing the car, sweeping the patio, painting the house, planting a garden, or taking the baby for a stroll — whatever physical activity you can think of to be done outdoors, do it. Even if it's only for ten minutes, it *will* make a difference. When done outside, even the chores won't seem like chores but investments in your health.

Any activity you do outside, even walking, increases your inhalation of fresh air. But realize that there is less oxygen in hot weather than in cold. That's why you are more alert and active on a crisp fall day than you are during a heat wave. Avoid exercising outside in any extreme weather: if

168 GREATER HEALTH-GOD'S WAY

it's too hot or too cold, stay inside. If you live in an area that has polluted air, stay inside on bad days and make doubly certain you are out soaking up the fresh air and sunshine on clear days.

You will have more benefits from all the other Seven Steps to Greater Health if you don't neglect this one. It's like the oil that keeps a machine running smoothly. You will experience more peace, digest food better, enjoy greater benefits from exercise, have an easier time of fasting, receive more cleansing from water, and sleep better at night if you make outdoor physical activity a way of life.

Learn to Breathe

In the exercise chapter, we talked about inhaling life and exhaling impurities. The life-giving oxygen that we inhale through the lungs is carried by the blood to all parts of the body and exchanged for carbon dioxide. Toxins in the body are released through this carbon dioxide. If a person does not get enough fresh air or is a shallow breather, there are certain poisons in the system that do not get out. In fact, one of the most important things that happen during exercise is what occurs throughout the entire body due to the deep breathing.

Life is more dependent on air than on anything else. Without it, death is only a few minutes away. The cleaner the air that you breathe, the better off you are. Breathing air that someone else has already breathed is very unhealthful, and gyms and exercise rooms that do not circulate fresh air are unhealthful. Avoid them and look for places that have good natural lighting—windows and skylights—and a way to circulate fresh air. Breathing stale air can cause nervousness, exhaustion, dizziness, sluggishness, and headaches.

Everyone should have "breathers" throughout the day. When you feel tired because the work you do requires more mental activity than physical, the exercise of deep breathing can do wonders. It can help you to relax, and also wake you up. It is a body balancer. Breathing deeply and slowly helps your entire nervous system. I've worked with dance instructors, speech therapists, singing teachers, and childbirth delivery coaches, and they have all taught me basically the same thing: to learn to breathe correctly. The basic "breather" they all taught consisted of these four steps:

1. **Inhale slowly to the count of five. As** you do expand your ribs, back, abdominal cavity, and lungs, so it is not just shallow breathing in the chest. You should be sitting or standing up straight and your shoulders and chest should not rise.

2. **Hold your breath for two counts.**

3. **Exhale slowly to the count of five** so that all air is gone.

4. **Hold for two counts and begin again.** Repeat five times.

It is best to breathe in through the nose and out through the mouth. The nose is equipped to filter and temper the air, making it perfect for your lungs, the mouth is not. You can breathe *out* through either the nose or the mouth.

Don't allow carbon dioxide to build up in your body. Every time you think of it during the day take a "breather." When you feel angry because someone cut in front of you on the freeway, or you're nervous about making a certain phone call, or the dentist is working on your lower molar, or you're running late, or you're waiting for an elevator, or you've been sitting in one place too long, or you're feeling groggy, take a breather. You'll find when you do, that you become refreshed, invigorated, calm, clear-minded, and more alive. You will also find that deep breathing during the day helps you to sleep better at night.

Do your best to see that the air you breathe is clean. Always ask for no-smoking sections on planes and in restaurants. If you're a smoker, get free of the habit immediately. Millions of people have done it, including me and my husband, so you can do it, too. It is an unnatural and unnecessary habit that does nothing good for you and only makes you smell bad, age prematurely, and die young. Breathing the smoke of *others* is very bad for you, too. Do all you can to avoid it. God did not create air filled with smoke. That, of course, is man's creation.

If you always remember that air is like food, you will be careful to get enough and get it as close to the way God made it as possible. Oxygen is a detoxifier. It removes poisons from the body and anything that does that lengthens life. If the waste thrown off by the lungs is retained, the blood becomes impure. Remember, dirty blood is a breeding ground for disease. So keep breathing!

How To Have a Healthful Wardrobe

Your skin breathes, too, and this is important to remember. We breathe through our lungs but we also breathe through our pores. *Wearing clothing that breathes is vital to good health.* I learned this from several nutritionists and it has had a life-changing effect on me. This may sound silly or unimportant, but when you wear one hundred percent man-made fibers there is a restriction of circulation and a depletion of energy. I have seen demonstrations of how certain man-made fabrics can sap your strength and energy when you wear them. Can't you honestly think of some outfits you've put on that were exhausting to wear? Perhaps they were too heavy or too tight — or sometimes it may have been that they had too many man-made fibers. This is something to consider.

Why let the clothes you wear restrict your life, your oxygen intake, or your energy? Try wearing loose-fitting cotton outfits for a week and see if you don't have more energy. I'm not saying you have to run out and throw away all your polyester shirts, I'm just saying that, as a way of life, wearing natural fibers is healthier. Once again, you don't have to be legalistic about it, just aware. When you have a choice, make it in favor of natural fibers if possible.

If you are feeling weak or rundown, consider wearing one hundred percent cotton outfits for a few days. I don't believe your body is tired *because* of your all-nylon dresses, but I do believe you can give a tired body a break by not wearing things that are exhausting. Test it for yourself. See if you don't have things in your closet that take more effort to wear than others. Try to balance them out. If you have an exhausting wardrobe, the next time you shop, try to buy something of cotton, silk, or wool—or maybe seventy percent cotton, for example. See if it doesn't make a difference. Especially in extreme weather conditions where temperature and humidity tax the body anyway. There is a lot to be said for God-made substances. Always buy clothes that allow your body to breathe and don't restrict your circulation. It is important to your health.

Balance, Balance, Balance

People develop different kinds of problems from too much sun and then blame it on the sun itself. Actually the problem is their own toxic body that couldn't handle the sun and their lack of wisdom as to how much sunshine they should get. God made man to be out in the sun. God also gave man enough sense to come out of it when it gets too hot. Some people go to extremes and bake in the sun, damaging their skin. Others look as if they've never seen the light of day because they do not go outside at all. Again there must be a balance. The rays of the sun give energy and life, but too much is destructive. Overexposure and sunburn are harmful and can cause a toxic reaction in the body. There are other health problems (not the least of which is skin cancer) that can occur from constant overexposure to the sun.

It's important to make a distinction between periods of fresh air and sunshine becoming a natural part of your life and lying in one position on the beach for hours and hours. I am not urging you to run a marathon on a hot smoggy day or to swim when it's snowing. I'm speaking of nice pleasant days with no extremes—be out there in them, enjoy them, and breathe in deeply. They are beautiful days that the Lord has made; rejoice and be glad in them.

When you go out in the sun, begin with short periods of time if you are not used to it: ten minutes in the spring and summer months and twenty minutes in fall and winter. Work up from there. The best rays of the sun are in early morning and late afternoon; after ten in the morning and until two in the afternoon the rays are the most intense and can be damaging. You can also damage your skin from too *long* an exposure to the sun. Sun yourself gradually, and in summer months always use a sun screen for protection. You will find that the better health you have the better you will tan—more evenly and more beautifully.

Once again I repeat, there must be a balance of all of the Seven Steps to Greater Health. This step might not seem as important as the others, but it is. Even when there is no sun, you can still get fresh air. Just be careful not to get chilled. Enjoy fair weather when you have it by getting outside and soaking up the fresh air and sunshine. When the weather is bad, concentrate on the other seven steps. Remember, there is a fine line between too little sun causing deterioration and a sickly constitution, and too much sun causing premature aging. Balance, balance, balance!

Fitting It Into Your Life

Like all of the other seven steps, getting enough fresh air and sunshine did not come naturally to me. I was never one to go outside, especially on a daily basis. I rarely saw the light of day through most of the year, and then in the summer I would bake, burn, and peel my skin in a matter of six weeks. When I first began to be aware of how God intended us to live in sunlight and clean fresh air, I had to write it into my schedule. That sounds absurd, I know, but I found that I wasn't the only one: many people in my classes had the same problem. It wasn't that they didn't want to do this step, they would just forget. So I started giving them a weekly schedule, and each day they had to spend ten to sixty minutes in the fresh air and sunshine. This helped them to establish new patterns of living and to break old habits. The same is true for you. You may have to write it into your schedule so that you will remember to spend ten to sixty minutes in the fresh air and sunshine every day. If you keep this and all the rest of the seven steps going strong for three months, you will have established some lifelong patterns of living that will keep you healthy, youthful, attractive, and alive. Once these become established habits, you don't have to think about them all the time. They become a way of life.

Do you live in a place that has windows and plenty of natural light? Can the windows be opened to allow fresh air to circulate? If not, make doubly sure that you take periodic outdoor breaks. If you don't have a backyard, pool, or nearby park, and if you don't feel safe walking around the block in your neighborhood, then at least open a window and sit in the sun and fresh air for a while as you read a book, polish your shoes, or do a few stretching exercises. If you live in a dark place with no fresh air and sunlight and where it's not safe to walk outdoors (and even if it were, the air outside is polluted), you should consider moving out of such an unhealthful environment into one more pleasant.

You would be surprised at how many headaches, bad attitudes, and even illnesses are caused by air pollution *in* the home. Be aware of the dangers of certain products, buy less-toxic products when you can, and keep your home well-ventilated when you use them. Check your home for air polluters. Things like bug spray, hair spray, room deodorizers, and bathroom cleaners can all add up to much irritation to your system. I realize they are important at certain times, but don't use them liberally or frequently.

If you ever feel yourself getting frustrated, irritable, or in need of a new attitude in general, try going for a walk outside in the fresh air and sunshine. You may come back in twenty minutes feeling like a new person. "No one can comprehend what goes on under the sun." [1]

All this may seem insignificant, but remember that EVERYTHING YOU DO COUNTS—whether it be something for good or something for evil; it will add up points for life or points for death. Whenever faced with a decision of any kind, no matter how small or insignificant it may seem, choose life! CHOOSE LIFE! Fresh air and sunshine are life giving.

[1] Ecclesiastes 8:17 (NIV)

Words of Truth

*"And God said, 'Let there be light,' and there was
light. God saw that the light was good, and
He separated the light from the darkness."*
Genesis 1:3 & 4 (NIV)

*"...So that from the rising of the sun to the place
of it's setting men may know there is none beside me.
I am the Lord, and there is no other.
I form the light and create darkness..."*
Isaiah 45:6-7 (NIV)

"Light is sweet, and it pleases the eyes to see the sun."
Ecclesiastes 11:7 (NIV)

*"Send forth your light and your truth,
and let them guide me."*
Psalm 43:3 (NIV)

"Even in darkness light dawns for the upright."
Psalm 112:4 (NIV)

*"I will put breath in you, and you will come to life.
Then you will know that I am the Lord."*
Ezekiel 37:6 (NIV)

*"Anyone who claims to be in the light but
hates his brother is still in the darkness."*
I John 2:9 (NIV)

CHAPTER 7

Step Seven: Perfect Rest

Everyone longs for, seeks after, and will go to great lengths
to achieve deep, sound, rejuvenating, refreshing sleep. But
those who have it on a regular basis are very few. Most of
us sleep restlessly, fitfully, shallowly, or on and off. The
hours we sleep may be too few, too many, odd, or unnatural.
We resort to tranquilizers, sleeping pills, alcohol, drugs,
television, or anything that will numb our minds, stop our
thought processes, and release us into mindless oblivion.
And still we wake up feeling as if we had never slept. Sleep
is a natural part of life and should come easy. Why doesn't
it? What is it exactly that keeps us tossing and turning?
Why is it so hard to stop thinking and wind down? Why
does a frontal lobotomy sometimes seem like the only
solution to this problem? The reason is because we are not
living the way God intended us to live during our waking
hours.

More Than a Good Mattress

Sleep is absolutely essential to good health and to life, and
for many people it is no problem. But for millions, sleep is
abnormal or irregular and some never sleep much at all. I
know what that's like because I suffered from insomnia for
years—from my preteens until just five years ago when
God showed me the Seven Steps to Greater Health and I
began applying them strictly to my own life. I found out
that if I ever neglected any one of the first six steps, my
sleep suffered. When I was totally at peace in every aspect

of my life (everything brought to the Lord daily); when I ate only food the way God made it; when I got plenty of exercise, fresh air, sunshine, and water; and when I fasted and prayed on a regular basis, I couldn't keep sleep from happening. You see, sleep is something that comes automatically to a healthy body.

There are other extremes, too. Some people sleep almost all the time. They seem to need fifteen hours of sleep a day and they get it in the classroom, at work, at parties, during a sermon, and even on the freeway. This tendency indicates there is something out of balance in the system. The Lord has given us a time to be awake and a time to sleep. A healthy body does not get confused about this. Most healthy people need only seven to nine hours of sleep in every twenty-four-hour period. Both extremes — too much or too little — are unbalanced and are signs that something in the lifestyle needs to be realigned.

Rest is the last of the Seven Steps to Greater Health, not because it is the least important, but because when all of the other steps are acknowledged and followed, restful sleep will be the automatic result. No straining, striving, conniving, or drugging will be necessary. In fact you will no longer need to be concerned about it, except for a few easy preparations or precautions.

No Substitutes

Many of you who read this book have been using drugs or alcohol on a regular basis as substitutes for sound restful sleep. If you are, go ahead and admit it. Bury your face in this book and say, "God, I confess that I use substitutes for the real thing on a regular basis." Don't say, "Who, me? A good Christian like me? An elder? A Sunday school teacher? Why, I give generously to my church, my children are in a good Christian school, I read the Bible, I pray, I'm a good person. Me?" Please! I am not accusing you of being a drug addict. In fact, I don't ever want to put you on the spot in this book. I just want you to examine yourself without any guilt or self-reproach, and invite you to live the way God intended you to live, to experience health and life the way He wants you to have it. However, you can't experience health and life if you regularly use substitutes for the real thing in *any* area of your life.

You see, the problem with using drugs, whether pain-killers, diet pills, or sedatives, is that you are merely hiding the problem. You are not making the problem go away — it's still there,, you're just masking it. While the problem is masked, you don't really know what's going on behind the mask. I don't mean to say that in extreme cases you can't take pain pills, tranquilizers, sleeping pills, or other medications prescribed by a doctor. I'm just saying that there is a danger in prescribing medicine or drugs for yourself on a regular basis. You always have to pay for every unnatural act you do in life, and somewhere down the line you will pay for it in your body as well as in your mind and spirit. There are enough tragedies that happen in life where you may need one of these "medical blessings." Don't misuse them by taking them as a way out of day-to-day problems. Don't allow drugs to become a way of life. If you always rely on aspirin or codeine to take your headache away without ever getting to the bottom of why you have headaches in the first place, how will you be able to take the steps necessary to eliminate the source of the problem. The same is true for sleep. The sleep you get with drugs is a sleep substitute and it's not the real thing. I grant you that a sleep substitute feels better than no sleep at all, but to use sleep substitutes as a way of life will slowly break down your body and mind and lead you to an early grave. You can and must be free of them. The way to do it is through the Seven Steps to Greater Health. Follow them all and keep them all in balance. You eventually won't need a single substitute in your life because you'll have the real thing.

Again let me stress that it is not my desire to make you feel guilty for using medication. For example, when you're in deep pain, take something. After all, pain can traumatize the body and perhaps do more damage than a pill could. Just don't make pills your way of life. See it as your goal to get well and be free of medication. Don't settle for *any* kind of substitute for the real thing *anywhere* in your life.

No Rest, No Life

Did you know that sleep is as necessary for survival as air, food, or water? Without air you can't live more than five minutes, without food more than ninety days, and without water more than a week. But if you were to not get any sleep for more than ten days, you would die. Nothing else will substitute for sleep.

I've heard people say, "I'm going to eat more today because I didn't get much sleep last night." It doesn't work that way. The two are not interchangeable. In fact, sleep is more vital than food. This was proven in an experiment by a medical professor, the results of which were published in a national magazine. This professor kept a litter of puppies awake for five days, at the end of which time they all died, even though they had been well-fed the whole time. While this was happening, another litter of puppies was allowed to have plenty of sleep but was not given any food for twenty days. At the end of that time the puppies were weak but they recovered totally when fed. These results are not surprising.

One dictionary defines sleep as "the unconscious state or condition regularly assumed by man and animals during which the activity of the nervous system is almost entirely suspended and the recuperation of the body takes place." During sleep food is transformed into tissue. A certain amount of time is needed to do that, and to rid the body of poisons. The cells in your body are repaired and reproduced more rapidly when you are sleeping than when you are awake and all the body functions are going at full speed. That is why there is no substitute for sleep. It actually changes the structure of the blood. There are certain things that need to happen in your body that can *only* happen during sleep. A tranquilizer helps you to go to sleep, but it interferes with some of the processes that need to happen in your body while you are sleeping.

Health, attractiveness, and beauty depend on good, deep sleep. Lack of sleep can probably age you more quickly than anything. And if you were unable to sleep at all for long enough, you would die. Wartime tortures include keeping victims awake to the point of insanity or near death, for then they can be programmed to do anything. We underestimate the powerful need for sleep and the destruction that happens in the body when we are deprived.

Sleep Stealers

Because the body rebuilds and repairs itself during sleep (especially the bloodstream) we must take great care to see that we get adequate sleep. Do you remember what I said about the necessity of keeping the bloodstream clean? Well, it can't happen without sleep.

One of the main causes for insomnia is *overeating* and *eating toxin-forming foods*. All items on the foods-to-avoid list are sleep stealers. When your body is full of toxic wastes, the nerves will be constantly irritated until the wastes have been eliminated. You will not be able to sleep well as long as the nerves are irritated. *Sleep is hindered if there are toxins in your body.*

Worry, fear, and *mental anxiety* are also sleep stealers. They keep you from falling asleep quickly and they wake you up in the middle of the night. If you are one of those who wakes up during the night and can't get back to sleep, check to see if you are repressing your problems instead of dealing with them. This will always hinder your rest. Psychological reasons for not sleeping should be taken up with the Lord immediately. Sleep is natural. God made you to sleep. Don't let yourself be deprived of it. Get to the bottom of what is keeping you from sleeping and take steps to see that it is corrected.

Those who sleep *too much* may also have too many toxins in the body or suffer from worry, fear, and mental anxiety. As you adopt the processes of natural living and reduce the amount of fatigue-causing poisons in the body, the craving for sleep is reduced.

Most victims of sleeplessness are those whose mental activity is much greater than their physical activity. When there is a lack of exercise and a diet deficient in anything — especially calcium — chances are you will not be resting as God intended you to rest. Remember what I said about how spending time in the sun aids calcium absorption? If you are not sleeping well at night, plenty of physical activity in the fresh air and sunshine might be the solution.

Too much noise, too much light, overcrowded sleeping conditions, restrictive clothing, not enough air or circulation, too hot a temperature, a mattress that is too hard, too soft, or too lumpy—all these will rob you of the sleep you need. Take steps to change anything that could be a sleep stealer.

Steps to Ensure Sound Sleep

Decide right now that good, healthful, deep, sound, refreshing, rejuvenating sleep is your natural God-given right. All you have to do is live the way God intended you to live. The following list offers suggestions that might help you if you're not sleeping as well as you should be:

1. **Go to bed early.** The dark hours before midnight are said to give you the most rest and do the most good. God made darkness for rest. It has been proven that the best sleep is obtained during those dark hours. Of course, I know this isn't always possible, but when you have a choice, make this your way of life. God didn't make us to stay up all night and sleep all day. You will find that you can sleep a solid eight hours from 9:00 PM to 5:00 AM and you will feel fresher and have more energy and clear-mindedness than if you sleep eight hours from 4:00 AM until noon. There is a quality of rest that happens in those evening hours before midnight. (If you are one of those people who is truly a night person, then the Lord must have called you to the "night watch" for a purpose and His grace will be sufficient for that.)

2. **Take mini-breaks during the day and rest totally for ten minutes.** You'll be surprised how this helps you to sleep better at night. If possible, take mini-breaks out in the fresh air and sunshine for even more benefits.

3. **Take frequent "breathers."** Doing the deep-breathing exercises that I mentioned in the preceding chapter

helps clean poisons from your system and calms your nerves.

4. **Increase your exercising.** Make sure your physical activity is as great as, or greater than, your mental activity. This also helps to flush out the poisons that irritate the nerves and cause insomnia.

5. **Get plenty of fresh air and sunshine.** Remember how you always feel like taking a nap when you come back from a day at the beach? All that vitamin D being manufactured when the sun hits your skin causes you to absorb calcium which soothes the nerves. If you consistently have problems sleeping, pay special attention to this step.

6. **Eat food the way God made it.** Natural foods, especially fresh fruit and vegetables, have a calming effect on the nerves. Keep your system free of sleep-disturbing poisons by eating God's food.

7. **Take a warm bath to relax.**

8. **Drink herb teas**—relaxing ones, like chamomile. Do not drink stimulants.

9. **Have a body massage or a foot rub.** Both are very soothing, healing, healthful, and conducive to good sleep.

10. **Fast and pray.** This will definitely help you to sleep better. While it may be true that sometimes you don't sleep as well during a fast as you would like, *after* the fast you will sleep better than ever because of the release of toxins from your system. Regular fasting is an aid to restful sleep.

11. **Take short naps.** A twenty- to thirty-minute nap during the day is effective, if you can train yourself to do it. You can't sleep well if you are overtired. (That sounds funny, but it's true.)

12. **Keep your sleeping room dark and quiet.** Too much noise and too much light interfere with sound rest.

13. **Buy a good mattress.** One that is not too hard, soft, or

lumpy. A good one is worth the price: it's an investment in your health and can affect your daily attitude.

14. **See that you have good ventilation.** It's important that your sleeping room isn't too hot, stuffy, or filled with unhealthful stale air. Too many people sleeping in one room is very unhealthy, also.

15. **Live in peace.** Because you will always rest more fully if you are at peace when you go to sleep, make the last thing that enters your mind before bedtime not some horror story on television, the terrors of a news report, a stimulating phone call, or an exciting book. Rather, have a short talk with God or read a few verses of His Word. If something is really heavy on your mind, get before the Lord and tell Him every detail. Don't take any of it to bed, but instead, leave it with God and sleep confident that you've covered the matter in prayer.

16. **Allow a half an hour to unwind.** I know this is a difficult step to do consistently if you are an extremely busy person and have a tight schedule, but if you can possibly work it out you will benefit greatly. Allowing a half an hour before bedtime to do *nothing* but unwind is a wonderful aid to a restful sleep. For example, if you must be up by 5:00 AM (perhaps in order to spend time with the Lord before the rest of the family is up at 6:00 AM), then you want to be asleep by 9:00 PM. So, from 8:30 PM to 9:00 PM plan to do nothing. Release the cares of the day, forget the project you're working on, and think of nothing that will keep your mind anxiously working all night. You can use this time to read the Bible or a soothing book of some sort, thumb through a magazine, take a leisurely bath, sit by the fire, watch something restful on television, get ready for bed, snuggle up with your mate, or whatever else comes to mind that would be a good way to end the day. The idea is to calm your spirit, mind, and body in order to prepare for a good night's rest from which you can wake up totally refreshed and ready to go the next morning.

17. **Have a nighttime ritual.** I'm told by psychologists that having a set habit of a few things you do before you go to bed helps prepare your mind and body for sleep. Something as simple as washing your face, brushing your teeth, combing your hair, covering the kids, putting out the cat, and padlocking the refrigerator will do it. Something to remember for all of life is that change wakes you up and habit puts you to sleep. See if you don't have some sort of simple routine that you do every night. Rejoice in those little nighttime habits and do not fear "rutdom" because they serve as signals to our body that you are shutting down for the evening and preparing for sleep.

18. **Remember the prayer closet.** If you do wake up in the middle of the night and you can't get back to sleep within thirty minutes, it is better to just get up and go talk to the Lord or read the Word than it is to lie awake the rest of the night and be angry about it the next morning.

19. **Check all of the Seven Steps to Greater Health** regularly. Remember that each one affects the others and all must be balanced. The automatic result of purifying your body through proper food, exercise, plenty of fresh air, sunshine, pure water, fasting, and prayer, in combination with a heart and mind totally at peace, is wonderful rejuvenating sleep. If all the steps are followed completely, sleep comes automatically and naturally. If you are not sleeping, check to see if one of the steps is out of balance.

20. **Don't wear restrictive clothing.** Wear clothing that is comfortable, loose, and made of materials that are not exhausting to wear.

21. **Under no circumstances drink alcohol, coffee, tea, or soft drinks and then take tranquilizers or sleeping pills.** Any one of these things alone is hard on your system. In combination they are deadly. Begin to see these things as ruled out of your new way of life. If your body is full of poisons of *any* kind, you cannot sleep soundly.

Cease From Your Labors

My husband and I had to be taught that vacations were not luxuries but spiritual necessities. Both of us have workaholic tendencies. We had to learn to balance work with *play*. We had to *learn* to cease from our labors and draw apart from the day-to-day world to spend time really resting. We had to be taught to take a vacation.

Vacations are important because we all need to stop our day-to-day work from time to time and relax and play for awhile. Allow your vacation to do that for you and don't make it burdensome. For example, driving nonstop for five days straight just to see the spot where General Snodgrass first spotted sharks in Alaska is not going to make you a healthier or a better person. It would be less work to stay home. Learn to rest.

I remember the first real vacation my husband and I took. It was not just a weekend away, but a two-week vacation in Hawaii. We arrived and checked into our hotel late in the evening so we had time only for dinner. Because of the time change we were up at five the next morning. We went jogging on the beach, swam in the ocean, played tennis, went horseback riding, snorkled, swam in the pool, ate a big breakfast — all before nine o'clock in the morning. We were two hyperactive workaholics from Los Angeles who, in the remaining thirteen days and twenty hours of our vacation, had to learn to relax, slow down, take it easy, lay back, and communicate. We had to *learn* how to *rest*.

Many people in the Bible, including Jesus, went away or drew apart from the world for a time of refreshing. You don't have to go to China to feel you've gotten away — you can do that one hour away from your home. The point is to get away and do something different — to experience a change of scenery and of lifestyle. If you live in the city, go to the beach, the lake, the country, the desert or the mountains. If you live a quiet life close to nature on a farm or ranch, perhaps you will want to go to the city, see the sights, and remind yourself of all that you are not missing.

Vacations are a good opportunity to enjoy God and His creation in a rich, full way — to meditate upon God and experience Him more fully. If you're a wife and mother, you may be asking yourself how you can experience God in a richer, fuller, uninterrupted way without leaving your husband and children at home and going on vacation by yourself. I admit that this is difficult, but it all depends upon the way you look at things. A time of uninterrupted communication with family members can be a form of communicating with God, too. God says, "Whatever you did for one of the least of these brothers of mine, you did for me."[1] When we minister to someone who needs us, like our husband or child, we minister to God, also. When we communicate on deep, meaningful levels with them, we have a spiritual experience.

Being away on vacation with your family gives you time to deepen your family ties and communication. There is a closeness that develops during that time together, and you have an opportunity to deal with things that need to be dealt with, such as unhealthy personality traits you see developing in children, misunderstandings that need to be cleared up, or a lack of communication that may have crept in unnoticed. You're all together in one car, one room, one plane, one tent, one table at a restaurant, and you see where you've failed to love, failed to discipline, failed to communicate, failed to understand, and you now have the opportunity to make those things right. The more time between vacations, the less time you've spent together at home, the more negligent you've been in dealing with problems, the more acutely these problems will show up on vacation. Don't be alarmed if they surface in the form of an argument or a "scene." This does not mean that the vacation is a total loss and you might as well go home. Be thankful these things are surfacing and take the opportunity to make things right and deepen your ties. It's a time of internal cleansing for the family.

You gain a new perspective on life when you get away. You see your life from a whole different viewpoint: you see what's out of balance, what you're doing wrong, and what you're doing *right*. You figure out what the "keepers" are in your life and what the "junk" is. Vacations help you to make clearer decisions about getting rid of the junk and

[1] Matthew 25:40 (NIV)

keeping the keepers. Remember, the first few days of any vacation are spent just winding down and changing your lifestyle, the second half is where the healing, growing, learning, communicating, and deep resting really happens.

Be aware of whether you are giving vacations their proper priority in your life. People who never take them end up taking their work and their day-to-day activities far too seriously. If you don't cease from your labors and allow yourself time to be refreshed and renewed, you will pay for it in your health and in your relationships with God and others.

Keep the Sabbath Day Holy

Time and time again the Bible mentions keeping the Sabbath Day holy and observing the principle of having one day of rest. Most of these Scriptures are in the Old Testament, the most well-known being in the Ten Commandments: "Remember the Sabbath Day by keeping it holy. Six days you shall labor and do all your work, but the seventh day is a Sabbath to the Lord your God." [2] God created this one day of rest and He gave it to man as a gift. "Bear in mind that the Lord has given you the Sabbath." [3]

Jesus said that He did not come to cancel the old laws: "Do not think that I came to destroy the Law or the Prophets, I did not come to destroy but to fulfill." [4]

An important part of the old law is the setting aside of one day for rest—a Sabbath Day. God knew that we would need a day to stop all that we do throughout the week and dedicate it to rest and refreshment in Him. It doesn't have to be Sunday, it could be any day. Many pastors take their Sabbath on Monday because for them Sunday certainly couldn't be called a day of rest.

If you work five days a week, use one of your days off for all errands, for "doing," and the other day for resting and seeking God, for "being." I don't want to suggest that this should become a legalistic burden. Let it become a freedom to move into. Your day of rest should be a day when you

[2] Exodus 20:8 (NIV)
[3] Exodus 16:29 (NIV)
[4] Matthew 5:17 (NKJ)

don't worry about the bills, your mind doesn't labor over your work project, you don't stop by the office, and you don't clean the house. You rest from all that you do throughout the week.

Once again, children and spouses are exempt. You can't get up in the morning and scream at your two-year-old, "Get your own breakfast! This is my day of rest!" This won't work. But you *can* have a different attitude about your duties. You can say, "This is my day of rest. I'm not going to worry about the missing button on the shirt, the spot on the carpet, the lawn that needs mowing, the report that's due next week, the deadline, the obligation, the phone call." Check out of the world and check in with God. He wants you to spend a day with Him, devoted to Him, being refreshed in Him. Read a book to His glory, take a nap, spend time together as a family. This is one day where you truly rest from all concerns and enjoy life, God, your friends, and family. The change from what you do during the week, plus a quiet time with God, helps to deeply refresh you and you'll find that you have much added strength for the other six days. It's one of God's wonderful ways, established for our benefit. If we obey this commandment and receive it like the gift that it is, we will have more peace and joy, and experience more fulfillment.

Entering Into God's Perfect Rest

The ultimate experience of God's rest will be when we have left this world and are with Him in heaven. The Scriptures say that people who doubt and disobey never enter His rest: "I said, 'They are a people whose hearts go astray, and they have not known my ways.' So I declared an oath in my anger. 'They shall never enter my rest.'"[5]

But God has promised those who love and serve Him that there is a rest for His people here on earth. We also know that there is *no* true peace or rest outside of His presence. "My presence will go with you and I will give you rest."[6]

[5] Psalm 95:10-11 (NIV)
[6] Exodus 33:14 (NIV)

We don't ever want to move away from the presence of the Lord so our prayer should always be the same as Moses' prayer when he said to God, "If your presence does not go with us, do not send us up from here." [7] In the presence of the Lord will be our true rest. "Come unto me, all who are weary and burdened, and I will give you rest. Take my yoke upon you and learn from me, for I am gentle and humble in heart, and you will find rest for your souls." [8] There is perfect rest when we surrender everything to God and link up totally with Him.

One of Bob Dylan's well-known songs says, "You gotta serve somebody. It may be the devil or it may be the Lord, but you gotta serve somebody." All of us are hooked up to something. Some people deny it—they sit with their cigarettes and Scotch on the rocks proclaiming they are free. We all cling to one thing or another—it's our nature. Anyone who says he is unattached is blind to his own attachments. We are like yoked oxen: whatever you are yoked with will eventually lead you around. When we are yoked with Jesus, He pulls most of the load and we just walk the path with Him. In being yoked with Him you will have perfect rest for your soul.

[7] Exodus 33:15 (NIV)
[8] Matthew 11:28-29 (NIV)

Words of Truth

"My soul finds rest in God alone."
Psalm 62:1 (NIV)

"I will lie down and sleep in peace, for You alone,
O Lord, make me dwell in safety."
Psalm 4:8 (NIV)

"There remains therefore a rest for the people of God."
Hebrews 4:9 (NKJ)

"My people will live in peaceful dwelling places,
in secure homes, in undisturbed places of rest."
Isaiah 32:18 (NIV)

"It is vain for you to rise up early, to sit up late,
to eat the bread of sorrows; for so He gives
His beloved sleep."
Psalm 127:2 (NKJ)

"This is the rest with which you may cause the
weary to rest."
Isaiah 28:12 (NKJ)

"For we who have believed do enter that rest."
Hebrews 4:3 (NKJ)

CHAPTER 8

Putting It All Together

We've come full circle in this book. We started out seeking peaceful living as the first step on the road to health and ended up with perfect rest as the final stage of living the way God intended us to live. Much more could be said about each of the topics dealt with in these chapters, and I hope what you read here will whet your appetite for more information on each subject. Now comes the question: "How do I put this all into practice in my life?"

Where Do I Begin?

You've read about all of the Seven Steps to Greater Health and it must seem a lot to remember. Much of it you may have heard before, but if you are not applying *all* of it to your life on a daily basis, then you are not enjoying the health, strength, and vitality that you could and should be enjoying.

There are times when everything seems difficult, especially when you are starting something new and changing some old entrenched habits. Changing old habits can seem a monumental task, but it's not. Jesus is always ready to help you. So you will have to put aside your fears and take the first step. If you believe that the Lord is telling you something about changing your ways, you should remember that God will never direct you to do anything unless He has prepared you to take the necessary steps. He wants you to live in *complete* health. God is on your side in this. He knows your battles and your weak points. If you're convinced that God is a good God and His ways are best, then just say, "Okay, God, let us together reorganize my life. I'm open to change. I know I need it. Show me what you want me to do."

Remember All of the Seven Steps

I don't want to bore you, but I must say once again that you must follow *all* of the Seven Steps to Greater Health. You cannot eliminate even one and have the others work. If you are not doing all of them, you are in for problems. You can say, "Oh, but I never drink water and I feel fine," or "I eat whatever I want and I don't get sick," or "I thrive on stress, it motivates me to bigger and better things," or "I don't have time for exercise; I have too many more important things to do," or "I've never fasted a day in my life and I don't intend to start now," or "I've gotten along all these years taking tranquilizers and I don't think they have a bad effect." But remember, heart attacks, strokes, cancer, and hundreds of other debilitating diseases don't give you a two-year warning so you can get your act together and go for a new body. They appear suddenly and often severely. They brew for a long time, and all of a sudden you wake up one morning with a pain, a lump, an inability to move, a weakness, or perhaps you don't wake up at all. Don't wait for the shocking jolt of awareness that you've gone too far doing your own thing. *Remember, no one is invincible or above God's laws.* Please care enough about God, yourself, and those who love you, to change your ways.

None of us are going to do all the steps perfectly. In fact, none of the seven steps came automatically to me. I had to learn them. I had to learn that I don't do well if I'm not exercising regularly. I had to learn how God intended us to eat. It was not easy for me to give up soft drinks and doughnuts for baked potatoes and steamed broccoli. I had to train myself to drink water by drinking it out of a measuring cup so that I would be sure that I was drinking enough. Being the food lover that I am, fasting certainly did not come easily to my nature. And even now I sometimes forget about fresh air and sunshine. I still battle with stress in my life. I constantly have to be on the lookout for signs that my schedule is becoming too full, that I'm trying to be super-woman, that I'm holding feelings in, that I'm listening to the wrong voice. I don't get sick or run down very often because I try to set limits, but when it does happen, the cause is no mystery. I can point right to the steps that I did not do. And I know exactly what to do to make things right again.

When one step is out of balance it throws all of the others off. For example, not getting enough rest for a few nights in a row will throw off your eating habits. You will either overeat to make up for how poorly you feel, or you'll crave junk food and won't have the strength to resist it. You won't feel good enough to exercise properly, you'll have a difficult time fasting, and you'll be so tired that you'll forget to drink water or go out in the fresh air and sunshine. You'll turn into a grump, alienate everyone around you, and end up with no peace of mind. This all happens because one—any one—of the steps was eliminated. Begin to be aware if one of the steps is slipping so you can head off problems before they happen.

Always keep in mind there is a fine line between grace (God does it), and obedience (I do my part). Doing it all by yourself is impossible. And if you cry "Grace!" over your sick, overweight body and then go have a chocolate dough-nut and a soda, that won't work either. There needs to be balance.

You must always begin by asking the Lord for every-thing. Ask Him to show you how you might have more peace and enter into His perfect rest. Ask Him to give you the discipline you need to exercise regularly. Ask Him to help you to lose interest in foods that are not good for you and to cultivate a desire and taste for those that are good. Ask Him to help you remember to drink water and to find time and ways to be in the fresh air and sunshine. Ask Him to make fasting an enjoyable, regular discipline in your life. He will certainly help you to do these things. They are His ways.

Next, you must do your part. And just remember that no matter how hard you try, there may come a time when you get a cold or flu or whatever. Don't torment yourself with thoughts of failure. Just calmly ask yourself if any of the seven steps are out of order. Have you let a couple go, or neglected some of the points under them? There is no doubt that Satan can attack you in your body, but we often make his job very easy. In fact, most of the time he doesn't do anything except tempt us and watch us do the rest ourselves. Because we have an uncanny way of forgetting about things that are good for us to do, it might be good from time to time to reread this book and to ask ourselves a few questions.

A Few Important Questions

Are you living in peace?

1. Are you spending time with the Lord daily in prayer?
2. Are you "'fessed up?"
3. Are you living with an attitude of praise?
4. Are you being fed by the Word of God each day?
5. Are you in touch with your feelings or are you holding things in and covering up your emotions?
6. Have you been careful to censor what comes out of your mouth? Have you been speaking life into your situations?
7. If you have deep emotional problems, have you sought the help of a counselor?
8. Are you denying something of your personhood by not being who you were created to be?
9. Has your life become too complex? Do you need to simplify?
10. Are you making choices for *life* every day?

Are you eating food the way God made it?

1. Are you eating food as pure as you can get it, or is processed food creeping into your diet?
2. Are you including fifty percent fruits and vegetables with every meal?
3. Have you kept red meat down to no more than two times a week, poultry two or three times a week, and fish two times a week?
4. Are you snacking on seeds, nuts, and berries?

5. Are you limiting dairy products and eggs to only three to four times a week?
6. Are you avoiding the foods on the foods-to-avoid list?
7. Are you including the foods on the foods-to-include list?
8. Are you careful not to gorge?
9. Have you kept your meals simple for the most part, or have they gotten too fancy?
10. Have you gotten into a diet rut where you are eating the same thing every day?
11. Are you careful to eliminate stressful situations during mealtimes?
12. Are you selective when eating out?
13. Are you following your doctor's orders?
14. Are you spacing your mealtimes five to six hours apart?
15. Are you careful not to have excesses or imbalances?
16. Have you been celebrating too many special occasions?

Are you getting enough exercise?

1. Do you have an attitude of activity?
2. Have you been consistent and regular in getting some form of daily exercise?
3. Are your exercises strenuous enough to force you to breathe deeply?
4. Are you walking every day?
5. Are you looking for ways to fit physical activity into your life?
6. Are you remembering that everything you do counts?
7. Are you refusing to listen to lies about yourself?
8. If you need to lose weight, are you burning more calories than you are taking in?
9. Do you remind yourself that physical exercise is a part of your ministry?
10. Do you remind yourself that you were not made to do nothing and that your body was meant to be used?

Are you drinking plenty of water?

1. Are you drinking six to eight glasses (sixty-four ounces) of water each day?
2. Are you avoiding coffee, tea, colas, and chemicalized fruit drinks?

3. Are you remembering not to drink anything one-half hour before meals and two hours after meals?
4. Are you drinking water that is pure?
5. Are you bathing regularly and using the loofa or dry brush?

Are you fasting and praying at least three or four days every month?

1. Are you remembering to pray while you fast?
2. Are you reading Isaiah 58 each time?
3. Are you getting at least sixty-four ounces of water during each twenty-four hours of fasting?
4. Are you controlling your food intake when coming off a fast (or are you making up for lost time?)
5. Are you remembering to break each fast with a raw fruit or vegetable?
6. Are you careful to see that you are going on carefully planned fasts and not just engaging in stop and start eating?

Are you getting enough fresh air and sunshine?

1. Are you spending time in surroundings that have an abundance of light and fresh air?
2. Are you remembering to do some form of physical activity outside for at least ten to twenty minutes each day?
3. Are you doing deep-breathing exercises every day?
4. Are you wearing "healthy" clothes or "exhausting" clothes?
5. Are you watching your time in the sunshine to see that you get neither too much nor too little?
6. Are you ignoring this step because it seems so insignificant and the others seem so much more important?

Are you getting plenty of rest?

1. Are you getting eight hours of sleep every night?
2. Are you allowing for a half hour to unwind before bedtime?
3. Are you staying away from chemical sleep inducers?
4. Are you getting to bed early enough in the evening?
5. Is it time for a vacation of some sort?
6. Have you been observing one day of rest every week?

Early Signs of Problems

In order to work with God to attain and maintain good health, we must keep our temple clean, well-nourished, and in good running order. Don't ever take God's grace and goodness for granted by ignoring signs your body gives you. Never overlook a plea from your body to change your ways. No matter how minor a signal seems to be, it is a sign that something is brewing and it could become serious if you don't make a change. Below is a list of early signs of problems that you should watch for. They are signs of a body that has a toxic buildup of some sort and they mean that one or more of the seven steps has been neglected. *Do not ignore any of these symptoms:*

1. white-coated tongue
2. constipation
3. frequent colds, stuffy nose, sneezing, sinusitis, sore throat
4. bad breath
5. body odor
6. overweight
7. underweight
8. fatigue
9. headaches
10. puffiness in the face
11. general aches and pains
12. nervousness, anxiety, or irritability
13. poor appetite
14. strong food cravings
15. cold hands or feet
16. anemia
17. dark circles under the eyes
18. sudden deepening of lines or wrinkles in the face
19. dry skin
20. oily skin
21. dry, flaking patches of skin around the nose, eyes, or mouth
22. pale, pasty complexion
23. skin breakout (pimples, boils, rashes, warts, etc.)
24. nails that crack, peel, or are brittle
25. any swelling, pressure, or soreness

26. menstrual problems
27. insomnia
28. digestive problems
29. bleeding gums
30. non-specific "crummy" feeling
31. painful, problematic feet
32. nausea
33. depression
34. poor posture
35. frequent sprains and pulls
36. sores in mouth
37. inability to concentrate or poor memory
38. hemorrhoids
39. poor sexual response
40. tender, rigid, or protruding stomach
41. listlessness
42. chronic boredom
43. high blood pressure
44. low blood pressure
45. blurred vision
46. looking older than your years, or suddenly looking older than you have been looking
47. constantly feeling cold or chilled
48. tight chest
49. frequent diarrhea
50. stiff joints
51. dull eyes
52. bloodshot eyes
53. burning, watering, or itching eyes
54. unsteadiness or weak muscles
55. drawn look in the face
56. hair lacking shine or body
57. hair breaking or falling out
58. hair too dry or too oily
59. feeling like you're headed for a mental breakdown
60. feeling as though life is out of control

To make sure that you are in order and moving with wisdom and obedience, at the first appearance of any of these signs, do these five steps:

1. **Take it to the Lord.** Tell Him your concern; pray for *total* healing.
2. **Ask God whether you should see a doctor.** If there is any doubt in your mind, go to the doctor.
3. **Ask God which doctor to see.**
4. **Ask God to give the doctor wisdom in treating you.**
5. **Ask God to give you wisdom in taking care of yourself.** If you feel clearly that your physical condition is *not* something you ought to see a doctor about, ask God how to get your body back in balance.

After you have taken these five steps, make any adjustments in your lifestyle necessary for your recovery, and pay strict attention to the Seven Steps to Greater Health. Whatever the problem is, get to the bottom of it before something worse happens. Don't think, "This is nothing, I can live with it." It may be true that you can live with it now, but can you live with it if it turns into something bigger? Watching for these early signs is a kind of preventative medicine.

Making It a Way of Life

In order to make the seven steps a way of life, you must be convinced that you need them. Then you must follow them consistently and long enough for them to become a habit. I got into this way of living because I was sick of being sick. It was very clear to me that the way I had been living was not working and that I needed to change. I am convinced now that these are God's ways and that they do work. That's why I obey them.

Do you know how good it feels never to have to worry about whether you're able to fit into your clothes when you need to go someplace? Of never panicking when the opportunity to go swimming arises and you're worried about whether you look presentable in a bathing suit? Or not to have your skin break out just before an important event? Or not to be sick when you need to be feeling your best? Or to have a body that's not going to give out on you when the going gets rough? *It feels wonderful!* Make God's ways your way of life and see for yourself. The only way to do that is to do these steps over and over and over until they become your new habits. Don't expect a lightning bolt to zap your taste buds, or your will. It rarely works that way, and it *never* works like that when God is trying to teach you a new way to walk. "No one ever hated his own body, but he feeds and cares for it."[1] "A man who strays from the path of understanding comes to rest in the company of the dead."[2] "Make level paths for your feet and take only ways that are firm. Do not swerve to the right or to the left; keep your foot from evil."[3] To make something a habit, you have to practice it over and over, every day. You have to fit it into your daily schedule.

Daily Schedule

I've asked you to give yourself three months of strictly following the Seven Steps to Greater Health before you judge the results. You will begin to see wonderful changes in your body the first week, but major improvements will come over a three-month period. It may seem time-consuming in the beginning but when these steps become a way of life, they will *save* you time. How do you weigh a little time spent each day against a few months in the hospital?

Many of you will face the problem I faced: these new ways may not come automatically. In that case, I suggest writing the steps into your daily schedule until they become second nature. This will give you a guideline as to what you are supposed to be doing. Don't leave it to chance or memory. Both are inadequate when it comes to dealing with something as important as your health. Once you learn balance and the right way of doing things, you won't need to chart your life. You'll have wisdom.

Buy a datebook with enough room to fill in ten to fifteen items under each day. Then fill in a week at a time with all that you need to do. (One day will be designated for fasting.) Eventually these things will be second nature and

[1] Ephesians 5:29 (NIV)
[2] Proverbs 21:16 (NIV)
[3] Proverbs 4:26-27 (NIV)

you won't have to be so strict about writing them down. Below is a sample daily schedule similar to the one I use in my classes. Make adjustments to fit your own needs.

Sample Daily Schedule

6:00	Wake up and drink two cups of water (or one cup of water and one cup of herb tea).
6:00-7:00	Spend time with the Lord in prayer, reading the Word, and worship.
7:00	Breakfast (includes fifty percent fruit).
8:00-9:00	Twenty to sixty minutes of exercise.
9:00-11:30	Sometime between two hours after breakfast and one-half hour before lunch drink two eight-ounce glasses of water.
12:00	Lunch (includes fifty percent vegetables or fruits).
2:00-5:30	Between lunch and dinner drink two glasses of water.
3:30-4:00	Time outside in fresh air and sunshine.
6:00	Dinner (includes fifty percent vegetables).
8:30	Two glasses of water before bedtime.
9:30	Stop whatever you are doing and begin winding down.
10:00	Bedtime.

Obedience is Better Than Sacrifice

If you're the type of person who doesn't want to sacrifice *or* obey then you do have a problem. If you look around you'll see people, individuals and groups, who are indulging their flesh with no limits and are paying for it in their bodies. Some have indulged themselves for so long that their spiritual eyes are now totally blind. They can't see the destruction they have brought upon themselves even as they are in the midst of it. But anyone who knows the truth ("He sent His word and healed them, and delivered them from their destructions."[4])—or better yet has the truth

4 Psalm 107:20 (NKJ)

living in him ("Jesus answered, 'I am the way and the truth
and the life.'" [5]) — has the advantage of being able to see the
right way. Such a person knows that a self-indulgent life
never brings fulfillment, but rather emptiness.

I believe that if you've come this far in this book you
already know this, and you *do* want to do the right thing.
The problem is we don't always see where we are not
obeying. We need always to question our actions: Are you
demanding healing from God for your arthritis, and yet
refusing to give up your coffee and cakes? Are you suffering
from chest pains and yet you will not slow down your busy
schedule? Are you mad at God because your back is out
again and yet you refuse to do the exercises the doctor gave
you? If you are not following your doctor's orders then you
are not being obedient. If you do not *trust* your doctor's
orders, then you need to re-evaluate what you are doing. If
you can honestly say that you believe your doctor's method
of treating you is wrong, then you should find another
doctor.

Just as you wouldn't have read this far unless you were
serious about your health and about obeying God, I am
certain that you will not finish this book without the Holy
Spirit convincing you of something you need to do. Don't
turn a deaf ear. We're talking about a lifetime of personal
freedom — the freedom to be who God created you to be in
Jesus, not a liberty to do whatever you want. It's the
freedom from the dictates of a worldly mind. Ask yourself:
"Am I willing to sacrifice something to walk in total
obedience to all the things the Lord is speaking to me
about?" Your obedience is important to God. He wants to
work through you and in you and He needs your coopera-
tion. Listen to Him. *Don't sacrifice your body to dis-
obedience.*

Don't ever envy people who don't know Jesus but seem to
have it altogether. They may have good health, great
wealth, and seem free of burdens. They say, "What do I
need God for?" Don't ever look at them and say to yourself,
"I'm being obedient for nothing. I see others who don't care
anything about God and are better off than I am." This is

[5] John 14:6 (NIV)

only an illusion. It is not the truth. In the Bible, David talked of that very thing. He looked at self-assured people and envied their prosperity: "They have no struggles; their bodies are healthy and strong. They are free from the burdens common to man; they are not plagued by human ills."[6] David couldn't make sense of that "Till I entered the sanctuary of God; then I understood their final destiny."[7] "How suddenly they are destroyed, completely swept away by terrors!"[8] Everyone eventually pays the price for not living God's way.

He Makes All Things New—And That Means You!

Always remember that in the Lord you go "from glory to glory,"[9] and "from strength to strength."[10] This means that if you seek after God and live for Him, *everything* that happens in your life is a step forward. This is true in your spiritual life as well as your physical body. It may seem at times that you are regressing, but this is not true. Some old bad habit may surface but this does not mean you are going backward, it means you are being given a new opportunity to learn to walk closer to God and see His power destroy it.

Always be willing to say, "Teach me your way, O Lord, and I will walk in your truth."[11] If you've got Jesus living in your heart, you've got everything you need to make it. By "making it" I don't mean acquiring a million dollars and having your picture on the cover of a national magazine. I mean having a life filled with purpose, peace, contentment, joy, and love. You're obviously a survivor or you would never have finished this book. Give yourself a break. Just because you learned some bad habits when you were younger, don't let them ruin your life now.

Jesus can set you free, and I know from experience that He is the *only* one who can. Let Him do it. Learn of His ways and follow them. It's worth the effort and so are you.

[6] Psalm 73:4-5 (NIV)
[7] Psalm 73:17 (NIV)
[8] Psalm 73:19 (NIV)
[9] II Corinthians 3:18 (NKJ)
[10] Psalm 84:7 (NKJ)
[11] Psalm 86:11 (NIV)

Again I say, *learn to love your body.* It is your friend, your helper, something to cherish, respect, appreciate, and applaud. It is not your enemy.

God redeems all things, restores all things, makes all things new — and that means your body. So don't be satisfied with feeling pain, fatigue, or depression. It is not God's plan for you to be sick or ailing. His plans for you are for good and not for evil. "'For I know the plans I have for you,' declares the Lord, 'plans to prosper you and not to harm you, plans to give you hope and a future.'" [12] God is on your side. God wants to renew all of you — your mind, your spirit, your health, your sex life, your work, your habits, your attitudes, your way of life. He makes *all* things new — and that means *you!*

Choose Life!

Balance is controlled living, but it is *not you* in control. It is *God* in control. That's the only way to achieve balance — allowing God to be in control of your life. "Show me the way I should go, for to you I lift up my soul." [13] Give every part of your life to God. Begin to see maintaining good health as a part of your ministry and service to Him.

God is the Giver of Life and the Healer, but He will always give *us* the *choice.* We are asked to choose what we want. Will you choose life? Will you choose death? "I have set before you life and death, blessings and curses. Now choose life." [14]

Remember: *Everything you do counts.* No matter how big or how small, whether it will count for good or for bad, *it will all add up.* Just make sure when it all adds up that you score at the top of the "good" column and at the bottom of the "bad." And don't be looking for shortcuts to good health. There aren't any.

The great Christian leaders, pastors, and teachers of our time agree that God is going to pour out His Holy Spirit over our land in a way we've never seen before. Powerful things are ahead. This is an exciting time to be living in.

[12] Jeremiah 29:11 (NIV)
[13] Psalm 143:8 (NIV)
[14] Deuteronomy 30:19 (NIV)

God is going to manifest Himself in a new way and He is going to do it through *you*. "Do you not know that you are the temple of God and that the Spirit of God dwells in you."[15] Make certain your temple is healthy, clean, and ready. Think how remorseful you'll feel if God knocks at your door and says, 'The time is now for you to do what I've created you to do. For such a time as this were you created. Rise up and go." And there you are, too sick to turn over in bed, let alone rise up and go.

We are partners with God. Do you know what it's like to be in a partnership with someone who is always sick and never shows up for work? The work is hindered. You have to find someone else to do the work and train them all over again.

When it comes down to the bottom line, however, there will be nothing more important than your relationship with God through Jesus—not even good health. Good health may fail and we may not be able to do everything right. But God will never fail. He is ours forever. "My flesh and my heart may fail, but God is the strength of my heart and my portion forever."[16] Even in dying we make choices: for eternal life or for endless suffering. Again I say, "Choose Life!"

[15] I Corinthians 3:16 (NKJ)
[16] Psalm 73:26 (NIV)

Words of Truth

*"He who listens to a life-giving rebuke will be
at home among the wise."*
Proverbs 15:31 (NIV)

"Whoever loves discipline loves knowledge."
Proverbs 12:1 (NIV)

*"I will not die but live, and will proclaim
what the Lord has done."*
Psalm 118:17 (NIV)

*"Beloved, I pray that you may prosper in all things
and be in health, just as your soul prospers."*
III John 2 (NKJ)

*"Blessed are all who fear the Lord, who walk in
His ways. You will eat the fruit of your labor;
blessings and prosperity will be yours."*
Psalm 128:1-2 (NIV)

"The Lord gives sight to the blind."
Psalm 146:8 (NIV)

*"Jesus Christ is the same yesterday and today
and forever."*
Hebrews 13:8 (NIV)

Recommended Reading

(These books are listed in the order in which each subject is dealt with in this book.)

1. Donsbach, Dr. Kurt, *Stress,* International Institute of Natural Health Sciences, Inc., Huntington Beach, CA, 1981.
2. Rinmer, Rosalind, *Prayer: Conversing With God,* Pyramid Books, New York, NY, 1973.
3. Allen, Charles L., *Prayer Changes Things,* Spire Books, Old Tappan, NJ, 1973.
4. Hayford, Jack, *Prayer is Invading the Impossible,* Logos International, Plainfield, NJ, 1977.
5. Bounds, E.M., *Power Through Prayer,* Zondervan Books, Grand Rapids, MI, 1972.
6. Seamands, David, *Healing for Damaged Emotions,* Victor Books, Wheaton, IL, 1973.
7. Littauer, Florence, *Blow Away the Black Clouds,* Harvest House, Eugene, OR, 1979.
8. LaHaye, Tim, *How to Win Over Depression,* Zondervan Publishing House, Grand Rapids, MI, 1974.
9. Cranor, Phoebe, *How Am I Supposed to Love Myself?,* Bethany Fellowship, Inc., Minneapolis, MN, 1979.
10. Hicks, Roy H., D.D., *He Who Laughs...Lasts and Lasts ....and Lasts...,* Hannuca House, Tulsa, OK, 1976.
11. Foster, Richard J., *Celebration of Discipline,* Harper and Row, San Francisco, CA, 1978.
12. Barnes, Emilie, *More Hours in My Day,* Harvest House, Eugene, OR, 1982.
13. Bonhoeffer, Dietrich, *The Cost of Discipleship,* Macmillan Publishing Co., Inc., New York, NY, 1979.
14. Kloss, Jethro, *Back to Eden,* Woodbridge Press Publishing Company, Santa Barbara, CA, 1975.
15. Jensen, D.C., Bernard, Nutritionist, *Survive This Day,* BiWorld Publishers, Inc., Provo, UT, 1976.
16. Jensen, Bernard, *Doctor-Patient Handbook,* BiWorld Publishers, Inc., Provo, UT, 1976.

17. Bragg, Paul C., *Building Health and Youthfulness,* Health Science, Dejent Hot Springs, CA, 1977.

18. Jensen, Dr. Bernard, *Nature Has a Remedy,* BiWorld Publishers, Inc., Provo, UT, 1978.

19. Heller, Dr. A.L., *Your Body His Temple,* Thomas Nelson Publishers, Nashville, TN, 1981.

20. Chapian, Marie, *Free To Be Thin,* Bethany House Publishers, Minneapolis, MN, 1979.

21. Cavanaugh, Joan, *More of Jesus, Less of Me,* Logos International, Plainfield, NJ, 1976.

22. Kuluinskaw, M.S., Viktoras, *Sprouts For the Love of Every Body,* O'Mango d' Press, Luethensfield, CT, 1978.

23. Forman, Ph.D., Robert, *How to Control Your Allergies,* Larchmont Books, New York, NY, 1979.

24. Turnbull, Yvonne, *The Living Cookbook,* Omega Publications, Medford, OR, 1982.

25. Turnbull, Bob and Yvonne, *Free To Be Fit,* Bethany House Publishers, Minneapolis, MN, 1982.

26. Chapian, Marie, *Fun To Be Fit,* Fleming H. Revel Co., Old Tappan, NY, 1974.

27. Donsbach, Dr. Kurt, *Drinking Water,* International Institue of Natural Health Sciences, Inc., Huntington Beach, CA, 1981.

28. Wallis, Arthur, *God's Chosen Fast,* Christian Literature Crusade, Ft. Washington, PA, 1974.

29. Smith, David R., *Fasting, A Neglected Discipline,* Christian Literature Crusade, Ft. Washington, PA, 1973.

30. Smith, J. Harold, *Fast Your Way to Health,* Thomas Nelson Publishers, Nashville, TN, 1975.

31. Cott, M.D., Allan, *Fasting: The Ultimate Diet,* Bantam Books, New York, NY, 1981.

32. Bragg, Paul C., *The Miracle of Fasting,* Health Science, Santa Barbara, CA, 1981.

33. Zamm, M.D., Alfred V., *Why Your House May Endanger Your Health,* Simon & Schuster, New York, NY, 1980.

34. McMillen, M.D., S.I., *None of These Diseases*, Fleming H. Revell Company, Old Tappan, NJ, 1983.